Orthodontics at a Glance

Orthodontics at a Glance

Daljit S. Gill

BDS (Hons), BSc (Hons), MSc, FDSRCS (Eng), MOrth,
FDS (Orth), RCS (Eng)

Consultant Orthodontist/Honorary Senior Lecturer
Eastman Dental Hospital (UCLH NHS Foundation Trust)/
UCL Eastman Dental Institute,
London, UK

Honorary Consultant Orthodontist
Great Ormond Street Hospital,
London, UK

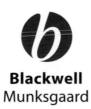

Blackwell
Munksgaard

Blackwell Publishing was acquired by John Wiley & Sons in February 2007. Blackwell's publishing programme has been merged with Wiley's global Scientific, Technical, and Medical business to form Wiley-Blackwell.

Registered office
John Wiley & Sons Ltd, The Atrium, Southern Gate, Chichester, West Sussex,
PO19 8SQ, United Kingdom

Editorial office
9600 Garsington Road, Oxford, OX4 2DQ, United Kingdom

For details of our global editorial offices, for customer services and for information about how to apply for permission to reuse the copyright material in this book please see our website at www.wiley.com/wiley-blackwell.

ISBN: 9781405127882

Library of Congress Cataloging-in-Publication Data
Gill, Daljit S.
    Orthodontics at a glance / Daljit S. Gill.
        p. ; cm. – (At a glance series)
    Includes index.
    ISBN-13: 978-1-4051-2788-2 (pbk. : alk. paper)
    ISBN-10: 1-4051-2788-0 (pbk. : alk. paper)   1. Orthodontics.   I. Title.   II. Series: At a glance series (Oxford, England)
    [DNLM: 1. Orthodontics–methods–Handbooks. WU 49 G475o 2008]

RK521.G55 2008
617.6′43–dc22   2007042412

A catalogue record for this book is available from the British Library.

Set in 9/11.5pt Times by Graphicraft Limited, Hong Kong
Printed and bound in Singapore by Markono Print Media Pte Ltd

6   2014

Contents

Acknowledgements and dedication

I would like to acknowledge the following people for permission to reprint figures used within the text:

Staff at the Eastman Dental Hospital (University College London Hospital NHS Foundation Trust, London)/University College London Eastman Dental Institute, London, and Farhad Naini (Consultant Orthodontist, St George's and Kingston Hospital), for providing some of the photographs used in this book.

Don Enlow and Mark Hans for Figures 3.1A, 4.1A, 4.1B and 4.1C.

Elsevier for Figures 5.1B and 35.1C (from Proffit, W.R. *Contemporary Orthodontics*).

Orthocare for permission to reprint the Dental Health and Aesthetic components of the Index of Orthodontic Treatment Need. The SCAN scale was first published in 1987 by the European Orthodontic Society (Evans, R. & Shaw, W. Preliminary evaluation of an illustrated scale for rating dental attractiveness. *European Journal of Orthodontics* 1987;**9**:314–318).

Dental Update for Figure 17.1B.

Dr Robin Richards (Department of Medical Physics and Bioengineering, University College London, London) for Figure 19.1D.

Finally, I would also like to acknowledge and thank Katrina Chandler and all the production team at Wiley-Blackwell for their enthusiasm, support and hard work throughout this project.

Dedication

I would like to dedicate this text to my parents and grandparents for the opportunities they have given me, their love, kindness and encouragement throughout my life.

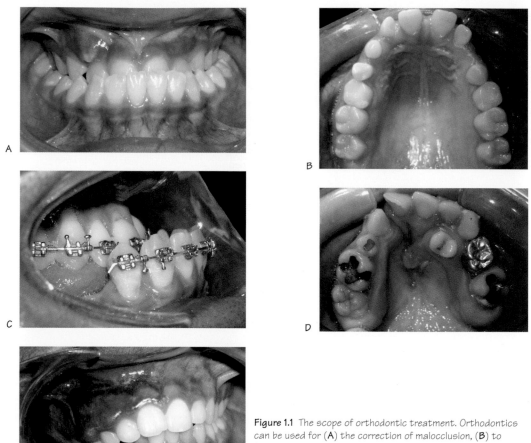

Figure 1.1 The scope of orthodontic treatment. Orthodontics can be used for (**A**) the correction of malocclusion, (**B**) to facilitate restorative treatment, (**C**) to aid surgical correction of severe skeletal discrepancies, (**D**) to facilitate the treatment of cleft lip and palate, and (**E**) for the comprehensive management of craniofacial deformity as in this patient with Sturge–Weber syndrome.

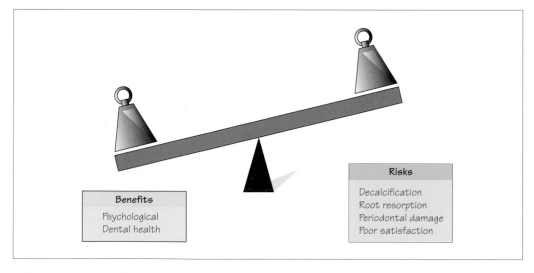

Figure 1.2 A risk–benefit analysis should be undertaken before commencing orthodontic treatment. Only if the benefits outweigh the risks should treatment be undertaken.

Orthodontics is the specialty of dentistry concerned with growth and development of the face and dentition, and the diagnosis, prevention and correction of dental and facial irregularities. The word orthodontics comes from the Greek words *ortho* meaning straight and *odons* meaning tooth.

The scope of orthodontic treatment

Orthodontic treatment is commonly undertaken for the management of malocclusion. Malocclusion is any deviation from normal or ideal occlusion. It should not be considered as a disease but a variation of normal. When such a deviation impacts on an individual's psychological or dental health one should consider orthodontic treatment.

Besides the management of malocclusion, orthodontics is increasingly being undertaken to enhance the results of other forms of dental and surgical treatment (multidisciplinary care, Figure 1.1A–E). For example, orthodontics can be used to facilitate:

- restorative treatment;
- the management of severe skeletal discrepancies in combination with orthognathic surgery;
- management of cleft lip and palate;
- management of severe craniofacial deformity;
- management of obstructive sleep apnoea.

The demand and need for orthodontic treatment

The patient's perception of the need for treatment does not necessarily always correspond with the professional's viewpoint. Often patients will request treatment when there is very little need on dental health grounds. In other cases, patients may not want to pursue treatment even when there would be a clear dental health benefit. A **risk–benefit analysis** is a useful method of determining whether to undertake treatment. This involves weighing up the risks and benefits of treatment and only undertaking care if the risks are clearly outweighed by the benefits (Figure 1.2).

The need for orthodontic treatment, based on professional criteria, is dependent on the population studied. The treatment need in the UK, on the basis of the Index of Orthodontic Treatment Need (IOTN, see Appendix 1), is estimated to be approximately 45% in 12-year-olds and 35% in 15-year-olds (IOTN Dental Health Component 4 and 5). The uptake of treatment among females is greater than among males even though the need is equal. In the USA, the treatment need is estimated to be 42% in white adolescents and 30% in black adolescents aged 12–17 years. These figures assume that patients who had already received treatment at the time of survey had a definite need for treatment.

Where is orthodontic treatment provided?

The majority of orthodontic treatment is undertaken within specialist orthodontic practices by orthodontic specialists or dentists with a special interest in orthodontics. The latter are not specialists but have undergone some training in orthodontics in addition to training at the undergraduate level. Hospital services provide treatment for those patients requiring complex multidisciplinary care and management of those malocclusions that are of value for the purposes of teaching and training. In the UK, the community dental services also provide care for people from disadvantaged groups for whom access to treatment is otherwise difficult.

How is orthodontic treatment provided?

The majority of orthodontic treatment is provided with the use of fixed orthodontic appliances. There has been a steady increase in the number of patients treated with fixed appliances over time (Table 1.1). The proportion of patients treated with removable appliances has reduced. The quality of the final occlusal result is significantly improved when fixed appliances are used instead of removable appliances. Removable appliances (e.g. functional appliances) are a useful adjunct to simplifying later fixed appliance treatment. The use of fixed appliances should not be attempted without undergoing comprehensive training.

Table 1.1 Types of appliance worn by 12-year-olds (15-year-olds) at the time of survey in 1993 and 2003 (data taken from UK Child Dental Health Survey).

	Percentage of 12(15)-year-olds wearing orthodontic appliances	
	1993	2003
Fixed	49% (68%)	72% (83%)
Removable	50% (37%)	28% (18%)

Craniofacial growth and development

An introduction to facial growth and development

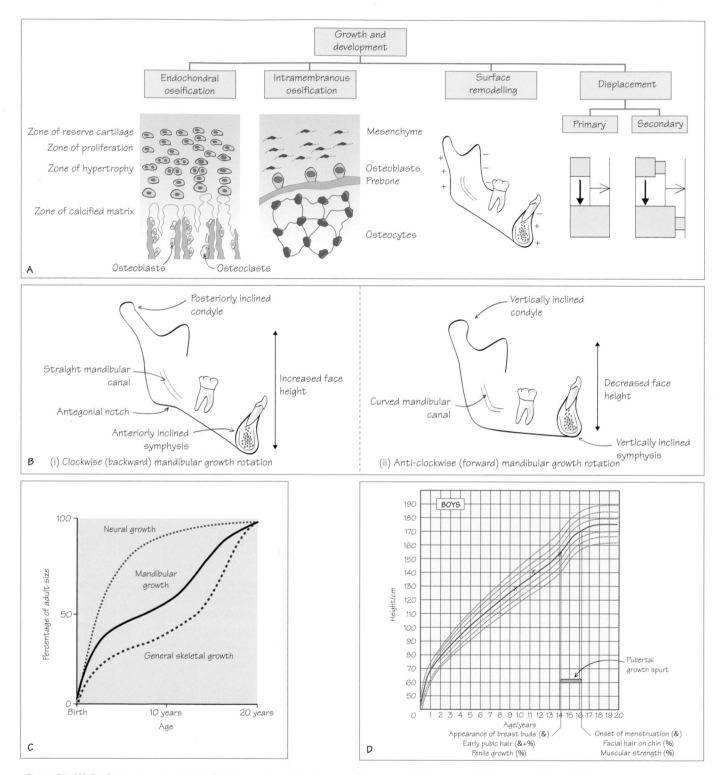

Figure 2.1 (**A**) The four main processes involved in growth and development of the craniofacial complex. (**B**) Various cephalometric features can indicate the likely direction of mandibular growth rotation. These features include the lower anterior face height, the shape of the lower border of the mandible, the inclination of the mental symphysis, inclination of the condylar head and curvature of the mandibular canal. (**C**) The general pattern of skeletal and neural growth is illustrated (Scammons curves). Mandibular growth has some similarity to the general skeletal growth pattern. (**D**) This figure shows the height curve for males. The average growth curve (50th centile) as well as curves between the 3rd and 97th centile are shown. The pubertal growth spurt is marked as well as the secondary sexual characteristics that may be present at the beginning and end of the spurt. At least three consecutive measurements (red crosses) are required to estimate with reasonable accuracy the growth curve any particular patient maybe following.

Facial growth and development is a complex three-dimensional process occurring until the late teens and then to a small extent in adulthood. **Growth** refers to an increase in tissue size as a result of cellular hypertrophy, hyperplasia, an increase in extracellular volume or a combination of these factors. **Development** refers to an increase in tissue organisation and specialisation. It is essential that the reader appreciates that there is tremendous **individual variation** in the *timing*, *magnitude* and *direction* of facial growth.

The importance of understanding facial growth

An understanding of normal facial growth and development is important to an orthodontist for several reasons:
- understanding the aetiology of malocclusion;
- recognition of abnormal growth patterns;
- treatment timing (e.g. functional appliances, orthognathic surgery);
- understanding factors influencing treatment stability.

Components of the skull

The skull can be divided into two main components:
- Neurocranium (cranial vault and cranial base);
- Viscerocranium (facial skeleton).

The **neurocranium** has an important role in supporting and protecting the brain, and provides a passageway for nerves and blood vessels. The **viscerocranium** is particularly important for mastication, respiration and supporting the eyes.

Processes involved in skeletal growth (Figure 2.1A)

Four processes are important during normal growth and development of the craniofacial skeleton:
- endochondral ossification;
- intramembranous ossification and sutural growth;
- surface remodelling;
- primary and secondary displacement.

Endochondral ossification is the process in which bone develops from a cartilaginous precursor. Cartilage is well adapted to undergoing compressive loading because of its avascular nature. Therefore, it is a good precursor in loaded areas such as the long bones, cranial base and mandibular condyle. **Intramembranous ossification** is a process in which bone is formed by osteoblasts present in mesenchymal tissue. It is an important mechanism of bone formation in non-weight-bearing areas such as the cranial vault, mandible and maxilla. **Surface remodelling** refers to the deposition and resorption of bone by the periosteum and endosteum. It alters the *shape* and *size* of individual bones and is important during growth and development of the entire facial skeleton. **Primary displacement** refers to the change in position of a bone by its own enlargement. **Secondary displacement** occurs when the position of a bone is changed because of growth of an adjacent attached bone. For example, growth of the cranial base has an important secondary displacing effect on the position of the maxilla.

The control of facial growth

Facial growth and development is dependent on the interplay between genetic potential and environmental influences. There has been much debate about which tissues have the genetic programming to control facial growth. The following have being suggested:

- bone;
- cartilage;
- soft tissues.

Many lines of evidence suggest it unlikely that osteoblasts and osteoclasts within **bone** hold the genetic programming to determine the *magnitude, direction* and *timing* of skeletal growth. Instead, it is accepted that the periosteum and sutures provide *adaptive* responses to external influences. Another popular theory is that the **cartilages** within the skull are the pacemakers of facial growth. It is suggested that the condylar cartilage and synchondroses grow to a genetically predetermined length and are replaced by bone, and thereby influence growth of the craniofacial skeleton. Experimental and clinical evidence indicates that growth of the **condylar cartilage** is not genetically predetermined, and like that of the sutures it is adaptive. In contrast, the **cranial base synchondroses** and the **nasal septal cartilage** have some genetic pre-programming that influences the magnitude of future growth. Growth of the cartilaginous nasal septum may be important for maxillary growth because it may place a downwards and forwards displacing force on the maxilla, creating tension across the maxillary sutures, leading to bone deposition and growth. The **functional matrix theory** suggests that the genetic control of facial growth resides in the **soft tissues** enveloping the craniofacial skeleton. The skull is said to consist of various skeletal units which are associated with a functional matrix whose activity determines the size, shape and position of the unit. Two types of functional matrix have been suggested:
- capsular matrices (e.g. neurocranial capsule, oro-naso-pharyngeal capsule);
- periosteal matrices (e.g. muscle and tendon attachments, teeth).

Growth of **capsular matrices** causes *displacement* of the associated skeletal units. For example, growth of the brain causes outward displacement of the cranial vault, and enlargement of the airway may lead to downward and forward displacement of the maxilla and mandible. Growth of the **periosteal matrices** is thought to influence the *size* and *shape* of the associated skeletal unit. For example, muscular pull and tooth eruption result in development of muscular processes (e.g. coronoid process) and the alveolar process, respectively.

Although the exact mechanism of facial growth control is not understood, current thinking supports the functional matrix theory and that some genetic control resides within the cranial base synchondroses and nasal septal cartilages.

Growth prediction

Because of tremendous individual variation, it is not possible to predict the *magnitude* and *direction* of future facial growth and chronological age cannot be used to predict the onset of the **adolescent growth spurt**. Some cephalometric features can help in predicting the likely direction of future mandibular growth rotations (Figure 2.1B), however, these are not entirely reliable. Concerning *timing*, mandibular growth follows the general body pattern of skeletal growth which accelerates at puberty (Figure 2.1C). Hence, serial **statural height** measurements and the presence of **secondary sexual characteristics** can help determine the onset and stage of the pubertal growth spurt and associated acceleration in mandibular growth (Figure 2.1D). This information can be helpful in timing the start of functional appliance treatment (see Chapter 39). The growth spurt that accompanies puberty can be expected at the age of **14 ± 2 years in boys** and **12 ± 2 years in girls**. The average duration of the growth spurt in boys and girls is 3.5 and 2 years, respectively. These figures are variable, both within and between populations.

3 Growth and development of the neurocranium

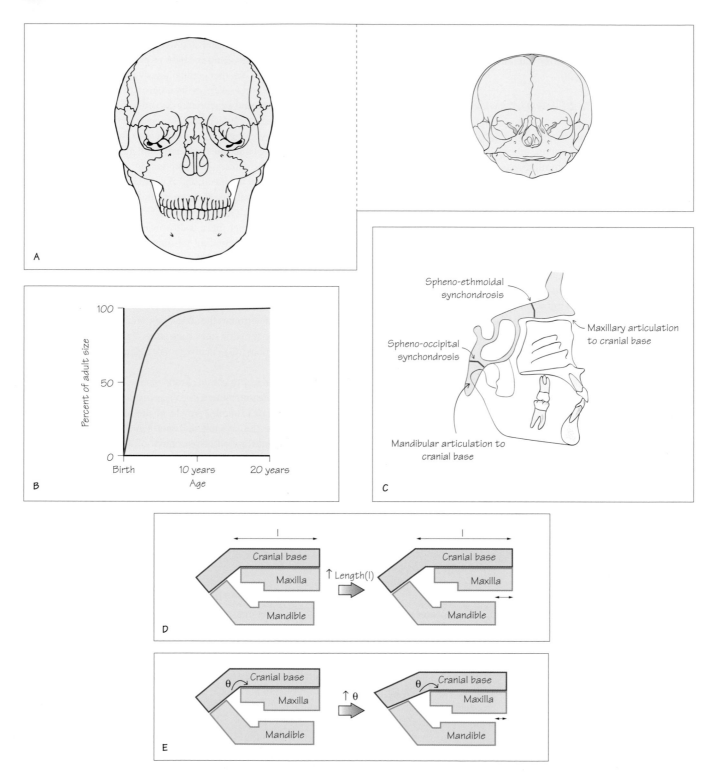

Figure 3.1 (**A**) In comparison to an adult skull, that of a new born child has a much larger cranial vault in proportion to the facial skeleton because of the relatively advanced neural growth. (**B**) A growth curve for the cranial vault. (**C**) The location of the main cranial base synchondroses and the relationship of these to the articulation of the maxilla and mandible. (**D**) The influence of cranial base length on the relationship between the maxilla and mandible. With an increase in cranial base length, there is a tendency towards a skeletal II pattern. When the length reduces, the skeletal pattern is likely to tend towards Class III. (**E**) The influence of cranial base angle on the skeletal relationship. With an increase in cranial base angle, there is a tendency towards a skeletal II pattern. When the angle reduces, the skeletal pattern is likely to tend towards a Class III relationship.

Cranial vault

The cranial vault is formed by the frontal, parietal, squamous part of the temporal and occipital bones. All these bones form by **intra-membranous ossification** of the mesenchymal tissue surrounding the developing brain, with centres of ossification first appearing at approximately **8 weeks** *in utero*. Sutures, which are periosteum-lined fibrous joints, separate the individual bones and provide tension-adapted growth. **Fontanelles** are found where sutures merge and increase the flexibility of the cranial vault to facilitate its passage through the birth canal during parturition. All the fontanelles are closed by the age of 18 months.

Growth of the cranial vault is largely determined by growth of the underlying brain. As brain growth is advanced at an early age, the cranial vault forms a major proportion of the skull in the newborn child (Figure 3.1A). The cranial vault achieves 90% of its adult size by the age of 5 years and nearly 100% by the age of 15 years (Figure 3.1B). After this, most changes occur due to enlargement of the frontal sinus and thickening of the anterior portion of the frontal bone. Important processes for normal cranial vault growth are:

• Sutural growth;
• Surface remodelling.

Expansion of the brain results in tension across the **cranial sutures**, which leads to bone deposition at these sites by intramembranous ossification. Therefore, sutures provide *adaptive* growth rather than having their own intrinsic growth potential. **Surface remodelling** also has an important role, with periosteal bone formation on the external surface of the cranial vault and bone resorption internally. As formation outpaces resorption, overall bone thickness increases during the period of active growth. The craniofacial bones become elevated into ridges by muscle pull and surface remodelling at sites of muscle attachment.

Cranial base

The cranial base provides the template for articulation of the maxilla and mandible, and its growth can influence the position and relationship of these bones. The cranial base begins development as several cartilages (the chondrocranium) which enlarge, fuse and undergo **endochondral** ossification at approximately **8 weeks** *in utero*. Bands of primary cartilage, known as synchondroses, remain where the individual cartilages fuse and have a significant role during growth (Figure 3.1C). The following synchondroses are particularly important:

• **Spheno-ethmoidal synchondroses** (grows until 6 years);
• **Spheno-occipital synchondroses** (grows until 13–15 years).

Important processes in cranial base growth include:

• Endochondral ossification;
• Surface remodelling.

The synchondroses provide pressure-adapted growth and consist of well-organised columns of cells (see Chapter 5, Condylar cartilage) aligned in the direction of future growth. They have a degree of intrinsic growth potential that results in the formation of new chondrocytes, their migration to the periphery, **endochondral ossification** and lengthening of the cranial base. The synchondroses contribute to cranial base growth until approximately 13–15 years of age. Following a decline in growth of the spheno-ethmoidal synchondrosis at the age of 6 years, the floor of the anterior cranial fossa becomes a stable radiographic structure on which sequential cephalometric radiographs can be superimposed to measure overall facial growth changes.

As the spheno-occipital synchondrosis is located between the anterior cranial fossa, to which the maxilla is attached, and the glenoid fossa, with which the mandible articulates, its growth has an important influence on the relationship between these bones (Figure 3.1C). For example, excessive growth can lead to an increase in **cranial base length** and development of a skeletal Class II relationship whereas deficient growth is more likely to result in a skeletal Class III relationship (Figure 3.1D). The morphology of the cranial base also influences the relationship between the mandible and maxilla. For example, a large **cranial base angle** (Figure 3.1E) can contribute to a skeletal Class II relationship whereas a reduced angle increases the likelihood of a skeletal Class III pattern.

Surface remodelling is important for increasing the size of the cranial fossae (the inner surface is resorptive and the outer is additive), maintaining the relationship between the foramina and an increase in the size of the sphenoidal and ethmoidal air sinuses.

Growth and development of the naso-maxillary complex

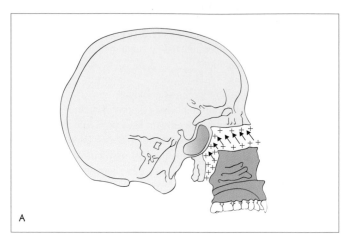

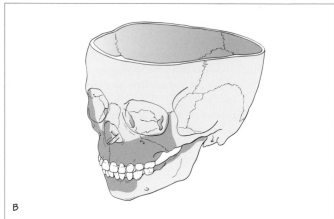

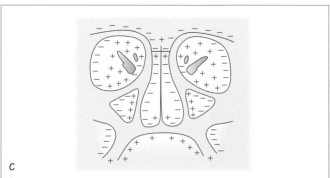

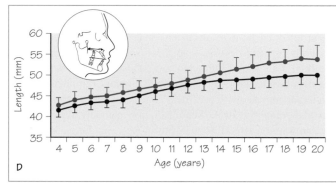

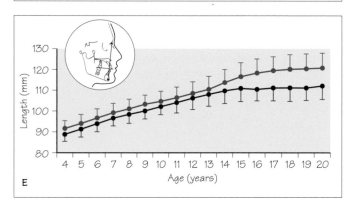

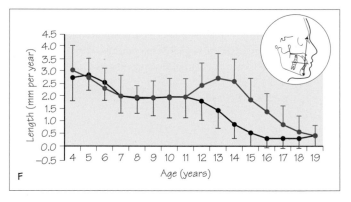

Figure 4.1 (**A**) Tension placed across the circum-maxillary sutures leads to bone deposition by intramembranous ossification and primary displacement of the maxilla. (**B**) Surface remodelling, by bone deposition and resorption can produce additive and substractive changes in the maxilla. The shaded areas are resorptive whereas the non-shaded areas are additive. (**C**) The palate descends as a result of growth due to surface remodelling. Bone is deposited on the oral aspect and resorbed from its nasal surface. This is responsible for an increase in the vertical size of the nasal cavity. +, areas of bone deposition; –, areas of bone resorption. (**D**) A distance curve for maxillary length showing the cumulative growth of the maxilla as a function of age. The blue line shows male and the magenta line female growth. The error bars represent the standard deviation of each mean value. Maxillary length was measured between ANS and PNS (see inset). (**E**) A distance curve for anterior facial height showing the cumulative growth in face height as a function of age. The blue line shows male and the magenta line female growth. The error bars represent the standard deviation of each mean value. Anterior face height was measured between nasion and menton (see inset). (**F**) A velocity curve for anterior facial height showing the average growth per year. The blue line shows male and the magenta line female growth. The error bars represent the standard deviation of each mean value. Anterior face height was measured between nasion and menton (see inset). Data for (D), (E), (F) taken from Bhatia and Leighton, 1993. A manual of facial growth. Oxford University Press.

The maxilla forms by **intramembranous ossification**, which first occurs within the maxillary process of the first pharyngeal arch at **8 weeks *in utero***. The maxilla is suspended from the undersurface of the anterior cranial fossa by the circum-maxillary sutures. The cartilaginous nasal septum, extending between the cranial base and nasal surface of the palate, is intimately related to the maxilla.

Implant studies show that on average the maxilla grows downwards and forwards from the anterior cranial base at approximately 50° to the sella–nasion line. However, there is tremendous *individual variation* with some having an almost horizontal, vertical or intermediate direction of growth.

Mechanism of maxillary growth

Processes involved in the growth of the maxilla include:
- Primary and secondary displacement;
- Intramembranous ossification;
- Surface remodelling.

As the maxilla is suspended from the cranial base, anteroposterior growth of the cranial base results in its **secondary displacement** (Figure 3.1D). This is an important mechanism contributing to anterior maxillary translation up to the age of 7 years when neural growth is largely complete. From this point, growth at the spheno-occipital synchondrosis, which continues until 13–15 years, can contribute up to 30% of total anterior maxillary movement.

Downwards and forwards movement of the maxilla is also associated with bone formation by **intramembranous ossification** at the circummaxillary sutures (**primary displacement**). The sutures have no intrinsic growth potential themselves but adapt by bone deposition to tension generated across them (Figure 4.1A). There is evidence that the **cartilaginous nasal septum** has some innate growth potential such that it places a downwards and forward force on the maxilla which creates tension across the circum-maxillary sutures. However, it is likely that the **functional matrices** also exert a significant anterior displacing force. Compressive ($\rightarrow\leftarrow$) or tensile ($\leftrightarrow$) forces can be placed across the sutures with headgear or protraction headgear, respectively. This can temporarily inhibit or potentiate bone formation at these sites, respectively. However, the original growth pattern will re-establish itself once this treatment ceases.

Bone formation at the **midpalatal suture**, particularly its posterior region, is an important mechanism for transverse maxillary growth. When transverse growth is active, one can expect <1 mm growth per year. Maxillary width reaches its adult dimensions by the age of 16 years.

Surface remodelling has a large influence on maxillary growth with bone resorption occurring on its anterior surface and bone deposition in the tuberosity region (Figure 4.1B). Growth at the maxillary tuberosity is an important mechanism contributing to an increase in arch length. Resorption on the anterior surface of the maxilla can negate the anterior movement produced by other mechanisms.

The palate descends by deposition on its oral surface and resorption on the nasal surface. This helps increase the vertical nasal dimension and size of the maxillary sinuses (Figure 4.1C). Eruption of the maxillary dentition and the associated alveolar development contribute significantly to vertical maxillary growth. Because the maxillary incisors are labially inclined and molars are buccally inclined, their eruption contributes to anteroposterior and transverse growth to a small extent, respectively. Transverse growth of the maxilla also occurs by surface deposition in the posterior buccal regions.

Timing of maxillary growth

Figure 4.1D shows a distance-growth curve for male and female maxillary growth measured as maxillary length, plotted against age. Maxillary growth begins to plateau at 16 years in males and 14 years in females. For the *average* individual, minimal growth changes can be expected after the age of 18 years in males and 17 years in females. The growth spurt associated with puberty is not as significant in the maxilla as in the mandible (see Chapter 5).

A comparison of Figures 4.1D and 5.1D shows that annual growth increments are greater in the mandible than the maxilla and that mandibular growth continues for a longer duration. This difference is termed **differential mandibular growth** and is important because, depending on the direction of growth, it can lead to an improvement in a skeletal II or deterioration in a skeletal III relationship. Differential mandibular growth also contributes to the development of late lower incisor crowding (see Chapter 41).

Figure 4.1E shows the distance-growth curve for total **anterior facial height**. In this dimension, growth tends to plateau in males by 19 years and females by 17 years. Figure 4.1F shows the corresponding velocity curve and the acceleration in vertical growth associated with puberty is particularly clear in males.

As a general rule, vertical maxillary growth continues longer than horizontal growth which in turn continues after transverse growth has ceased.

Maxillary growth rotations

Growth rotations of the maxilla are not as significant as those in the mandible (see Chapter 5). The maxilla undergoes a small clockwise (backward) or anti-clockwise (forward) internal rotation during growth. This is compensated by varying degrees of bone resorption and deposition on the palate, such that there is normally little change in the inclination of the palatal plane, and tooth eruption (external rotation, see Chapter 5). The maxilla also rotates in the transverse dimension because posterior midpalatal growth exceeds anterior growth. This is responsible for a gradual reduction in arch length with age.

Post-adolescent maxillary growth

Research indicates that facial growth continues, although to a small extent, into adulthood. The pattern of growth is a continuation of the earlier changes. Generally, vertical growth predominates followed in reducing magnitude by changes in the anteroposterior and transverse dimension. Between the ages of 17 and 80 years, the magnitude of increase in maxillary length and lower anterior face height is in the order of 1 mm and 2 mm, respectively.

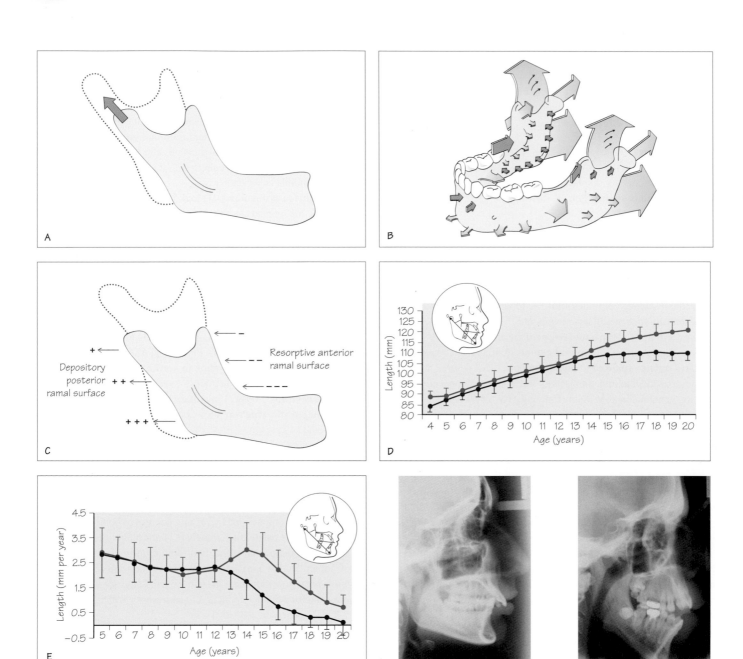

Figure 5.1 (**A**) The mandibular condyle is thought to respond to the downwards and forwards displacing forces exerted by the functional matrices with upwards and backwards growth by endochondral ossification. This results in primary displacement of the mandible. (**B**) The mandible undergoes significant surface remodelling during growth. Blue arrows indicate sites of resorption and red arrows indicate sites of deposition. (**C**) Surface remodelling results in uprighting of the mandibular ramus. The posterior ramal surface is depository whilst its anterior surface is resorptive. Different degrees of resorption and depositon occur along each surface resulting in ramus uprighting. (**D**) A distance curve for mandibular length showing the cumulative growth of the mandible as a function of age. (**E**) A velocity curve for mandibular growth showing the average growth per year. For (D) and (E) the blue line shows male and the magenta line female growth. The error bars respresent the standard deviation of each mean value. Mandibular growth was measured between condylion (Cd) and gnathion (Gn) (see inset). Data taken from Bhatia and Leighton, 1993. *A manual of facial growth*. Oxford University Press. (**F**) An example of extreme (i) anti-clockwise (forward) and (ii) clockwise (backward) mandibular growth rotation. Note the differences in the lower anterior facial height, overbite, chin prominence and lower incisor inclination.

The mandible forms by **intramembranous ossification**, which first occurs within the mandibular process of the first pharyngeal arch at **6 weeks** *in utero*. The mandibular condyles articulate with the glenoid fossae, which lie on the inferior aspect of the middle cranial fossa. The mandible grows downwards and forwards from the cranial base, with the vector of growth varying from a more horizontal to more vertical pattern among individuals.

Mechanisms of mandibular growth

Processes involved in the growth of the mandible include:
- Endochondral ossification;
- Surface remodelling;
- Primary and secondary displacement.

The condylar cartilage is a secondary cartilage that differs histologically from the cranial base synchondroses. It provides a pressure-resistant articular surface with multidirectional **adaptive growth** occurring by **endochondral ossification**. The condyle usually grows in an upwards and backwards direction (mean = 6° to the posterior border of the ramus), however, this can vary within and between individuals from a more backward to vertical pathway. It is thought that the condylar cartilage reacts by adaptive growth to the downwards and forwards displacement of the mandible caused by the **functional matrices** (Figure 5.1A). In some individuals, there is unequal growth of the two condyles, resulting in mandibular asymmetry.

Surface remodelling is important for the relocation of the rami in a posterior direction and lengthening the mandibular body by several centimetres, which helps accommodate the developing dentition. Generally, the anterior surface of the ramus is resorptive whereas its posterior surface is additive (Figure 5.1B). Differences in the magnitude of bone resorption and deposition result in uprighting of the ramus with growth (Figure 5.1C). The chin becomes more prominent with growth, especially in males following puberty, due to surface resorption above the chin point and bone deposition on the chin point. The muscular processes of the mandible (e.g. coronoid process, the angle) develop as a result of the activity of the attached musculature. Dental eruption leads to development of the alveolar process.

As the mandible increases in size it undergoes **primary displacement** in a downwards and forwards direction. In many individuals, the glenoid fossa remodels downwards and backwards with growth which causes downward and backward **secondary displacement** of the mandible. This partially counteracts the increase in chin prominence created by primary displacement. Vertical growth of the middle cranial fossa can also cause secondary displacement of the mandible by influencing the vertical position of the glenoid fossae.

Timing of mandibular growth

Figure 5.1D shows a distance-growth curve for male and female mandibular growth, measured as mandibular length, plotted against age. Mandibular growth begins to plateau at 18 years in males and 16 years in females. For the average individual, minimal growth changes can be expected after the age of 19 years in males and 17 years in females. The velocity-growth curve for male and female mandibular growth (Figure 5.1E) shows the annual growth increments plotted against age. The acceleration of growth associated with puberty in both males and females is seen clearly on this graph. However, the mandibular growth spurt in males is larger than that in females. Both the rate and duration of mandibular growth is greater than in the maxilla. **Differential mandibular growth** can have a number of clinical consequences (page 11).

As a general rule, vertical mandibular growth continues longer than anteroposterior growth, which in turn continues after transverse growth has ceased.

Mandibular growth rotations

Longitudinal cephalometric **implant studies** show that the mandible rotates as it grows downwards and forwards. Mandibular growth rotations result from a mismatch between growth in ramus height (posterior facial height) and lower anterior facial height (LAFH). There are two types of mandibular growth rotation:
- Internal rotation;
- External rotation.

The mandible can be viewed as consisting of an *internal* core of bone surrounding the inferior alveolar canal and an *external* surface comprising the periosteal surfaces and the erupting dentition. In most individuals, the internal core rotates in a anti-clockwise (or forwards) direction by an average of 15° between childhood and adulthood. However, the mandibular plane angle only reduces by ≤5° during this period as the external mandibular surfaces compensate for the internal rotation by selective surface resorption, deposition and tooth eruption. Effectively, on average 15° of anti-clockwise (forwards) internal rotation is compensated by 10° of clockwise (backwards) external rotation.

Great **individual variation** exists in the pattern of rotation described above. Internal rotation may occur to a greater than normal extent or may even occur in a clockwise direction. If these changes are not compensated for adequately by external rotation, excessive rotation of the mandible result with a number of clinical consequences. These include:
- **Short face height (Figure 5.1Fi)** if there is excessive anti-clockwise rotation of the mandible. This results in reduced LAFH, prominence of the chin point and a deep overbite as the incisors rotate towards the palate.
- **Long face height (Figure 5.1Fii)** if there is excessive clockwise rotation of the mandible. This results in increased LAFH, reduced lip competence, reduced prominence of the chin point and a reduction in overbite or anterior open bite.
- **Altered chin prominence**. Clockwise mandibular rotation tends to decrease the prominence of the chin point whereas anti-clockwise rotation increases its prominence.
- **An altered path of incisor eruption**. Clockwise mandibular rotation generates a more anterior path of incisor eruption whereas anti-clockwise rotation establishes a more upright path. Incisor uprighting results in a reduction in arch length and precipitates incisor crowding (see **late incisor crowding**, see Chapter 41). Clockwise mandibular rotation results in the lower incisors being pushed into the lower lip, and consequent incisor uprighting and crowding.
- **Relapse of orthodontic treatment**. Clockwise rotation of the mandible results in downwards and backwards rotation of the incisors with a consequent relapse of anterior open bite and overjet correction. Anti-clockwise rotation can result in relapse of deep overbite correction.

Post-adolescent mandibular growth

As with maxillary growth (see Chapter 4), mandibular growth also continues into adulthood. Between 17 and 80 years mandibular length can increase up to 3 mm. Females tend to show a clockwise growth rotation whereas this rotation occurs in the opposite direction in males.

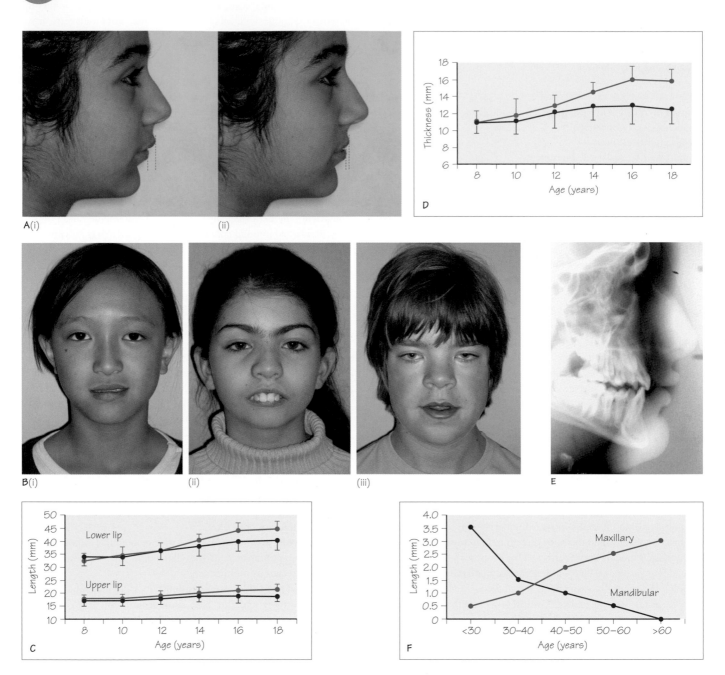

Figure 6.1 (A) Simulation effects of upper incisor retraction on the upper lip. Comparison of the pre-treatment (i) and post-treatment (ii) photographs shows that the upper lip is less prominent after 4–5 mm of upper incisor retraction. (B) The upper lip length is measured between subnasale and stomium superius. (i) Normal upper lip length; (ii) short upper lip length – note the increased upper incisor display; (iii) long upper lip – note the reduced upper incisor display at rest. (C) Changes in upper and lower lip length with growth. The blue lines represent male changes and magenta lines corresponding female changes. The error bars represent the standard deviation of the mean changes. Data taken from Mamandras A.H. (1988) *AJODO* **94**(5): 405–10. (D) Changes in upper lip thickness with growth. The blue lines represent male changes and the magenta line corresponding female changes. The error bars represent the standard deviation of the mean changes. Data is taken from Mamandras A.H. (1988). *AJODO* **94**(5): 405–10. (E) The thickness of the soft tissues overlying the chin can contribute to a prominent chin point. In this example the soft tissue chin thickness in increased. (F) Graph to show changes in maxillary (blue line) and mandibular (magenta line) incisor exposure at rest, in relation to age. There is a gradual reduction in upper incisor exposure and increase in lower incisor exposure with ageing.

The soft tissues of the face influence facial appearance and the stability of orthodontic treatment. Anteroposterior movement of the incisors can alter lip position and impact on facial aesthetics (Figure 6.1A). Examination of the soft tissues during orthodontic assessment and knowledge of normal soft tissue changes during growth is important in planning the final position of the incisors and predicting the stability of treatment changes.

Growth in lip length

The upper lip length, measured from the junction between the base of the nose and the upper lip (subnasale) to the lowest point on the upper lip (stomion superius), should be 20–22 mm in adult females and 22–24 mm in adult males (Figure 6.1B).

The upper and lower lips continue to grow in length during adolescence with males having greater growth than females (Figure 6.1C). Growth of the upper lip, in males and females, tends to plateau at 18 years and 14 years, respectively. Vertical growth of the lower lip plateaus in both sexes at 16 years of age and exceeds growth in the upper lip. Because vertical growth of the lips exceeds vertical skeletal growth, the lips become more competent with growth *unless* there is an abnormal skeletal or soft tissue growth pattern. Therefore, incompetent lips at 8–10 years in many children may show self-correction with growth. Lip competency is an important factor in determining the stability of overjet correction following maxillary incisor retraction.

Growth in lip thickness

The thickness of the lips influences their fullness, which is an important factor in determining facial aesthetics. The relationship between the lips, nose and chin is particularly important in this regard. This can be assessed by judging the anteroposterior position of the lips in relationship to the E-line (see Chapter 15). The thickness of the lips also influences their likely response to incisor retraction. Thin lips are more likely to become more retrusive following incisor movement than thick lips as they are less self-supporting.

Growth in maxillary and mandibular lip thickness tends to plateau by the age of 16 years in both males and females. Thereafter, the lips, particularly the upper lip, tend to thin (Figure 6.1D). The normal upper lip thickness, measured cephalometrically from just below A-point, is 12–15 mm in Caucasians. The thickness is greater in people of African Caribbean origin.

Nasal growth

An understanding of nasal growth is important because it affects the *relative* prominence of the lips. The nose grows in a downwards and forwards direction with vertical growth exceeding anteroposterior growth. Overall, there is a greater increase in nasal dimensions in males than in females, and the adolescent spurt in nasal growth is more pronounced in males. Therefore, when assessing the relative prominence of the lips in a 12-year-old child, one would expect a greater reduction in prominence due to nasal growth in a boy than in a girl. Therefore, in young patients in whom the lips are retrusive, incisor retraction may be more damaging to male than female faces.

Growth of the chin

As well as nasal growth, growth of the chin can influence the relative prominence of the lips. The position of the chin is determined by the prominence of the bony mental protuberance and the thickness of overlying soft tissues (Figure 6.1E). Between the ages of 7 and 17 years, the normal increase in thickness of the soft tissues is small (approximately 1.5–2.5 mm). Therefore, in the majority of individuals, growth and development of the mandible is the primary factor affecting chin prominence. The normal soft tissue chin thickness is 10–12 mm in Caucasian adults.

Facial ageing

It is important to understand the soft tissue changes that occur with facial ageing. These must be considered during treatment planning to ensure that the incisors are not positioned so that they artificially age the patient. Some of the relevant changes that occur with ageing are listed below.

• A reduction in upper incisor show and increase in lower incisor show at rest (Figure 6.1F). This is due to sagging of the upper lip with age and toothwear. The ideal upper incisor show at rest is 2–4 mm with females showing more than males. Incisor movements that increase tooth display include retraction and extrusion. Movements reducing incisor display include proclination and intrusion. The effect of such movements on incisor display must be considered during orthodontic treatment planning so as not to artificially age a patient.

• The lips become less prominent. This is due to thinning and sagging of the soft tissues. In borderline cases, these changes can be exacerbated by inappropriate incisor retraction during earlier orthodontic treatment.

• The maxillary incisors tend to upright.

• The nose becomes more prominent and the nasal tip descends. Increased nasal prominence exacerbates reduced lip prominence.

• The vertical height of the vermillion reduces and the commissures drop.

• Deepening of the nasolabial folds.

7 Development of the dentition

Table 7.1 Calcification and eruption dates of the primary dentition. The mandibular tooth in any series usually erupts before the maxillary counterpart. Root formation is usually complete 12–18 months after eruption.

Eruptive sequence	Calcification begins (*in utero*)	Eruption
Central incisors	12–16 weeks	6–7 months
Lateral incisors	13–16 weeks	7–8 months
First molars	14–17 weeks	12–15 months
Canines	15–18 weeks	18–20 months
Second molars	16–23 weeks	24–36 months

Table 7.2 The second deciduous molars can have various occlusal relationships: distal step; flush terminal plane; or mesial step.

Second deciduous molar relationship	Prevalence
Distal step (i)	10%
Flush terminal plane (ii)	30%
Mesial step (iii)	60%

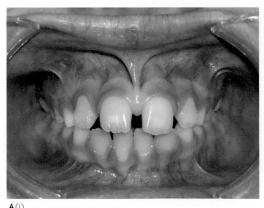

(i) (ii) (iii)

Table 7.3 Calcification and eruption dates of the permanent dentition. Root formation is usually complete 24–36 months after eruption.

Eruptive sequence	Calcification begins (months)	Eruption (years)
First molars	Birth	5–6
Mandibular central incisors	3–4	6–7
Maxillary central and mandibular lateral incisors	3–4	7–8
Maxillary lateral incisors	10–12	8–9
Mandibular canines	4–5	9–10
Maxillary first premolars	18–21	10–11
Mandibuar first premolars	21–24	10–12
Maxillary canines	4–5	11–12
Maxillary second premolars	24–27	10–12
Mandibular second premolars	27–30	11–12
Second molars	30–36	12–13
Third molars	80–120	17–25

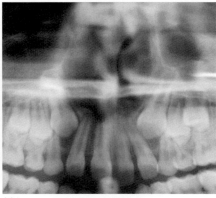

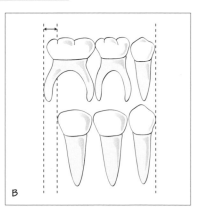

A(i) (ii)

Figure 7.1 (A) The ugly duckling stage of dental development: (i) the maxillary lateral incisors are distally splayed and there is a midline diastema; (ii) the radiograph shows that the distal splaying is due to pressure on the lateral incisor roots by the developing canines. (B) The combined mesio-distal width of the deciduous canine, first molar and second molar is greater than the combined width of the permanent canine, first and second premolar. The difference is termed the Leeway space.

Teeth develop from the **dental lamina** with first evidence of formation at **6–7 weeks** *in utero*. The stages of tooth development can be sub-divided into bud, cap and bell stages.

It is important to remember that dental age correlates poorly with chronological age and knowledge of the **normal sequence** of eruption is more important in detecting disturbances.

The primary dentition

The timing of calcification, eruption and root completion of the primary dentition is outlined in Table 7.1. Occasionally, a **natal tooth** is present at birth which is a prematurely erupted tooth of the normal series (usu-ally an incisor) or a supplemental tooth. These may have to be extracted if they cause problems with breast feeding or their increased mobility poses risk of aspiration.

Emergence of the primary dentition normally commences at 6–7 months with eruption of the lower central incisors closely followed by the remaining incisors. Compared to the permanent dentition, the deciduous incisors erupt relatively upright and spaced. Spacing further increases with growth of the alveolus. The first molars erupt at 12–15 months followed by the canines (18–20 months) and second molars (24–36 months). Because the lower second molar is wider than the upper, these teeth usually occlude with a flush distal surface, however, alternative arrange-ments can exist depending on the molar relationship (Table 7.2).

Spacing is particularly noticeable distal to the maxillary lateral incisors and mandibular canines. These are referred to as the **primate spaces** as many primate species have these throughout life. With age, the deciduous dentition can undergo significant toothwear, which encourages the development of an edge-to-edge incisor relationship.

Eruption of permanent teeth

Eruption of permanent teeth can be divided into four stages:
• **Pre-emergent eruption**. Eruptive movements begin at the com-mencement of root development. For eruption to occur, the dental follicle must resorb the overlying bone, or primary tooth root, and the eruptive mechanism should cause tooth movement. Normally both these mechanisms are coordinated, however if they are not, failure of eruption may result.
• **Post-emergent eruption**. Tooth eruption normally occurs when root formation is three-quarters complete. Eruption is rapid (0.3–0.5 mm/week) until the tooth reaches close to the occlusal plane (**post-emergent spurt**). Factors opposing eruption include occlusal contacts and pressure from the tongue and cheeks.
• **Juvenile occlusal equilibration**. Once a tooth has moved into occlusion, eruption continues at a slower rate to keep pace with vertical skeletal growth. This occurs as long as eruptive capacity is not exceeded. There is a spurt in eruption that coincides with the adolescent spurt in facial growth (see Figure 4.1F).
• **Adult occlusal equilibration**. This stage starts after the adolescent growth spurt. Teeth continue to erupt throughout adult life to com-pensate for occlusal wear and small increments of vertical skeletal growth. Overeruption can also occur if an opposing occlusal contact is lost. In total, the juvenile and adult occlusal equilibration phases account for approximately half the total tooth movement occurring during all the eruptive stages.

Mixed dentition

The timing of calcification, eruption and root completion of the perman-ent dentition is outlined in Table 7.3. The **early mixed dentition** com-mences with eruption of the lower central incisors and lower and upper first molars at approximately 6 years. The direction of eruption of the lower molars is at approximately 90° to the mandibular plane, and they are guided into position by the distal surface of the second deciduous molars. If these occlude normally, with flush distal surfaces, the first molars erupt into a half-unit Class II relationship (see Table 10.1). If there is spacing between the mandibular deciduous molars, this may close due to mesial pressure placed by the erupting first molar. This will result in mesial migration of the first permanent molar (termed **early mesial shift**) which may help towards establishing a Class I molar relationship.

The direction of eruption of the incisors is dependent on soft tissue factors, habits, and the direction of jaw rotation (see Chapter 5). It is normal for the incisors to erupt slightly lingual to their predecessors to reflect their developmental position. The maxillary central incisors and mandibular lateral incisors erupt at approximately 7 years. The maxil-lary central incisors may be distally inclined, with a diastema, as a result of pressure exerted on their roots by the developing lateral incisors. The maxillary lateral incisors erupt at 8–9 years and as they develop in a palatal position, the existence of crowding can result in palatal trapping. Because of pressure exerted from the developing canine, the lateral incisor may also be distally inclined. This is a normal stage of devel-opment which has commonly been termed the **ugly duckling stage** (Figure 7.1A).

As the permanent incisors are larger than the deciduous predecessors, the additional space for their eruption comes from a number of sources:
• spacing present between the deciduous incisors;
• an increase in arch circumference as the permanent incisors are proclined relative to their predecessors;
• an increase in intercanine width as the canines erupt occlusally *and* outwards. In addition, the lower canine erupts distally into the primate space.

It is normal for there to be a small amount of crowding (1–2 mm) of the lower incisors until the lower canines erupt. This is termed the **incisor liability** and can resolve following the increase in intercanine distance that follows canine eruption. More severe crowding is likely to persist.

The **late mixed dentition** commences with eruption of the mandibu-lar canine, mandibular first premolar and maxillary first premolar at approximately 11 years. The maxillary canines and second premolars erupt at approximately 12 years and are closely followed by the second molars. The maxillary canines develop high in the maxilla and migrate labially with development. They should be palpable high in the buccal sulcus at the age of 8–10 years. They erupt *after* the upper first pre-molars which increases their likelihood of being crowded. As the canines erupt the distal splaying of the incisors usually self corrects and any *small* diastema (<4 mm) will close. The third molars often erupt any time between 17 and 25 years if there is adequate space.

The combined width of the deciduous canines, first molars and sec-ond molars is greater than the width of the permanent canines, first and second premolars. The difference, termed the **leeway space** (Figure 7.1B), is greater in the lower (2.5 mm per side) than the upper arch (1.5 mm per side) due to the larger size of the lower second deciduous molars. The leeway space allows mesial migration of the first molar (termed **late mesial shift**), when the deciduous teeth exfoliate, with greater move-ment of the lower than the upper. If this occurs in combination with favourable mandibular growth, a Class I molar relationship is estab-lished in cases where a flush terminal or distal step relationship existed between the first deciduous molars (Table 7.2).

Archform

The dimensions of the dental arches continue to alter following dental eruption. In the **mandibular arch**, the intercanine width increases by 3–4 mm between 3 and 13 years. Following the eruption of the permanent mandibular canines, this dimension decreases by a mean of 1–2 mm up to the age of 45 years. The mandibular first permanent inter-molar distance increases slightly (1–2 mm) between 8 and 13 years and decreases minimally (~1 mm) thereafter.

In the **maxillary arch**, the intercanine width increases by 3–4 mm between 3 and 13 years. It continues to increase by 1–2 mm following eruption of the permanent canine until the age of approximately 45 years. The maxillary inter-molar distance shows a similar pattern of change as in the lower arch.

Diagnosis and treatment planning

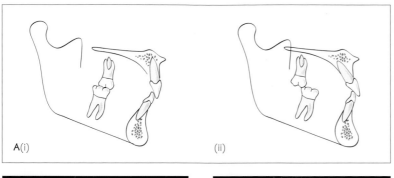

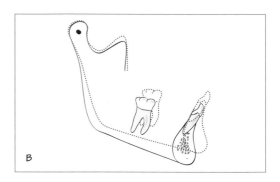

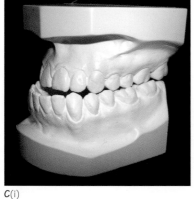

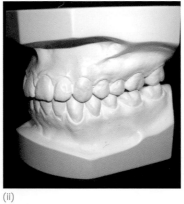

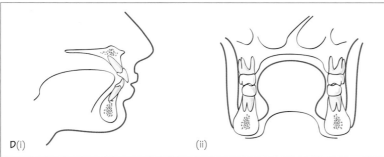

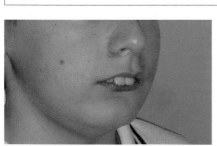

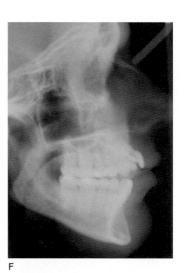

Figure 8.1 (**A**) Dento-alveolar compensation. Under the influence of favourable soft tissues, in Class II malocclusions (i) the lower incisors may be proclined and the uppers retroclined, and in Class III malocclusions (ii) the upper incisors may be proclined and the lowers retroclined to compensate for the sagittal skeletal discrepancy. (**B**) Interaction between the anteroposterior and vertical dimensions. Downwards and backwards rotation of the mandible results in a reduction of chin prominence. (**C**) The interaction between the anteroposterior and transverse dimension. Before treatment (i) there is a bilateral buccal crossbite. Treatment involving maxillary advancement (ii) has resulted in spontaneous correction of the crossbite as a wider part of the maxilla has been moved forwards relative to the mandible. This is an example of a relative transverse maxillary discrepancy. (**D**) Light, prolonged, resting forces placed by the lips, cheeks and tongue determine the position of the dental crowns above their apical base (equilibrium theory). (**E**) An example of a lower lip trap where the lower lip is trapped behind the upper incisors at rest. This can result in upper incisor proclination and retroclination of the lower incisors. (**F**) Anterior tongue posture. The tongue is clearly seen protruding between the insisors and making contact with the lips at rest. This may have contributed to the development of the increased curve of Spee in the upper arch and the anterior open bite.

An understanding of the aetiology of malocclusion is important in the prevention and stable correction of occlusal discrepancies. Malocclusion is due to a combination of **genetic**, or inherited, and **environmental** factors. The relative importance of each of these depends on the trait under examination. From a clinical perspective, it is useful to classify the aetiology of malocclusion under the following headings: skeletal factors; soft tissue factors; dento-alveolar or local factors; and habits.

Some of these factors are inter-related, for example the skeletal pattern can influence lip position. Commonly the aetiology of malocclusion is **multifactorial**.

Skeletal factors

Skeletal factors should be considered in three planes.

Anteroposterior

The anteroposterior (AP) relationship of the maxilla and mandible can have a large influence on the sagittal occlusal relationship. If the soft tissues are favourable, the incisors may compensate, by proclination or retroclination, for a given skeletal discrepancy. This is termed **dento-alveolar compensation** (Figure 8.1A). In such cases, the occlusal discrepancy will appear less severe than the underlying skeletal defect. If the soft tissues are unfavourable, the malocclusion may appear worse than the underlying skeletal discrepancy. For example, a lower lip trap can exacerbate a Class II malocclusion by causing upper incisor proclination and lower incisor retroclination.

A **skeletal II** pattern commonly arises due to mandibular retrognathia but can also result from maxillary protrusion. Mandibular retrognathia may be due to reduced mandibular length, a posteriorly placed glenoid fossa and/or an abnormality of the cranial base (see Figures 3.1D, 3.1E). The vertical dimension can also influence the AP position of the chin point. For example, if the vertical dimension is increased, due to downwards and backwards rotation of the mandible, the chin point will also rotate backwards (Figure 8.1B).

A **skeletal III** pattern may be due to maxillary retrusion and/or mandibular protrusion. Again the defect may lie within the individual jaw bones or at the level of the cranial base.

Vertical

The face height influences the overbite, lip competency, the lower lip line and the AP position of the chin.

Growth rotations of the mandible (page 13) are responsible for the development of abnormalities in facial height. An extreme clockwise (backwards) or anti-clockwise (forwards) rotation can result in a long and short face, respectively.

Excessive vertical growth of the maxilla (**vertical maxillary excess**) results in an increase in face height and chin point retrusion by causing downwards and backwards rotation of the mandible.

Transverse

Ideally, the maxilla should be slightly wider than a corresponding point on the mandible to produce the normal buccal overjet of 2–4 mm. In those with maxillary retrusion, the maxilla is often reduced in size in all three dimensions such that a transverse deficiency also exists. This is termed an **absolute transverse maxillary deficiency**. As the sagittal and transverse dimensions are inter-related, an AP discrepancy between the maxilla and mandible can also result in a transverse mal-relationship (**relative transverse maxillary discrepancy**) even when the absolute width of the maxilla is normal (Figure 8.1C).

Dento-alveolar compensation, by *buccal* upper molar and *lingual* lower molar tipping can compensate for transverse maxillary

deficiency. In such cases, the occlusal discrepancy may not appear as severe as the underlying skeletal defect.

Soft tissue factors

The teeth lie in a position of muscular balance determined by **prolonged and light resting forces** placed by the lips and cheeks on the outside and the tongue on the inside (**equilibrium theory**) (Figure 8.1D). Forces generated by the periodontal ligament may also contribute to this equilibrium.

The **fullness and tone of the lips** has an influence on labiolingual incisor positioning. When the lips lack muscular tone and are flaccid, the incisors tend to be proclined. When the lips are tense, the incisors maybe retroclined. The term **strap-like lips** is used for highly active lip musculature.

The **lower lip line** is the vertical relationship between the lower lip and the maxillary incisors in the rest position. Ideally, the lower lip should cover one-third to one-half of the upper incisor crowns. When the coverage is greater, the upper incisors may be retroclined, and when reduced the incisors may be proclined.

Lip competency, the lower lip line and the method used to obtain an **anterior oral seal** are inter-related. When minimal muscular effort is required to achieve an oral seal, the lips are termed competent. The term **lip incompetence** is used when excessive muscular activity is required to achieve an oral seal. Incompetent lips are often associated with a *low* lower lip line. With incompetent lips, it may be possible to produce an anterior oral seal by excessive mentalis activity or forward mandibular posturing. If it is not possible to produce a seal by these mechanisms, the following **adaptive swallowing patterns** may exist:

- Tongue to lower lip;
- Lower lip to palate;
- Tongue to upper lip.

An anterior tongue position, as in a tongue to lower lip seal, may result in incisor proclination. A lower lip to palatal seal (Figure 8.1E), results in upper incisor proclination and lower incisor retroclination. A tongue to upper lip seal, sometimes seen in Class III malocclusions, can produce upper incisor proclination.

The size, position and function of the **tongue** may influence dental development. **Macroglossia** and an **anterior tongue position** (Figure 8.1F) may impede incisor eruption and lead to the development of an anterior open bite. The effects of an atypical swallowing pattern, where the tongue is involved in the formation of an anterior oral seal, has been mentioned above. Rarely, a neuromuscular defect may lead to an **endogenous tongue thrust** where the tongue is forcibly thrust forward during swallowing. This can result in incisor proclination and the formation of an anterior open bite.

Enlarged **adenoids** have been implicated in anterior open bite development. It is suggested that enlargement results in increased resistance to nasal airflow and mouth breathing. With constant mouth opening, the molars overerupt, the face height increases, and an anterior open bite develops. There is insufficient evidence to recommend early removal of enlarged adenoids to prevent occlusal problems.

Patients with **generalised pathology of muscle** (e.g. muscular dystrophy) maybe more prone to an increased vertical dimension and anterior open bite. A reduction in the force of contraction of the muscles of mastication, at rest and during function, may lead to excessive vertical skeletal growth and molar overeruption.

Patients with muscle weakness due to generalised pathology of muscle may be more prone to molar overeruption, increased vertical growth and anterior open bite (Table 13.4, Figure 26.1Aiii).

The aetiology of malocclusion: (ii) locals factors and habits

Table 9.1 The effects of early loss of deciduous teeth. Balancing extraction refers to the loss of teeth from the contralateral side of the arch to minimise a centreline shift.

Tooth lost	Effects on permanent dentition	Action required
Deciduous incisors	• Minimal effect – some space loss if crowding. Spacing may affect aesthetics	• None
Deciduous canines	• Centreline shift if unilateral loss with some relief of incisor crowding • Space loss for permanent canines	• If crowding, consider balancing extractions to protect the centreline
Deciduous first molars	• Small centreline shift if crowding with minimal relief of labial segment crowding • Mesial molar movement with space loss	• Consider balancing or space maintenance
Deciduous second molars	• Often no effect on centrelines or incisor crowding • Mesial drift of molars with space loss for second premolars	• Space maintenance except in spaced arches

Table 9.2 Consequences of infraocclusion of a deciduous molar.

Tooth	Consequences
Infra-occluded deciduous molar	• Delayed exfoliation • Progressive submergence with failure of alveolar development • Difficult extraction often requiring surgery
Permanent successor	• Delayed and abnormal eruption • Disturbed root development • Centreline shift
Developing occlusion	• Tipping of adjacent teeth • Localised posterior open bite • Higher frequency of canine impaction, hypodontia and ectopic first permanent molar eruption possibly due to a common aetiologic machanism

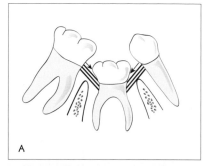

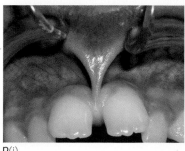

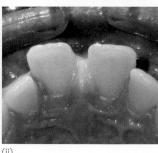

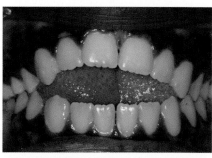

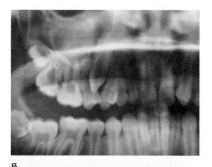

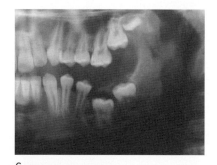

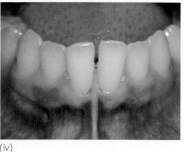

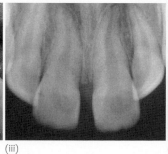

Figure 9.1 (**A**) Tension arises in the transseptal fibres (shown in red) as the infraoccluded molar moves below the occlusal plane. The direction of this force results in exaggerated tipping, reduced vertical development and a centreline shift of adjacent teeth. (**B**) Transposition of the right maxillary canine and first premolar. (**C**) Primary failure of eruption of the lower left first permanent molar. (**D**) (i) A low maxillary frenal attachment associated with a diastema. (ii) A positive blanch test. (iii) A small alveolar notch between the central incisors that results in disruption of the transseptal fibres. (iv) A high lower frenal attachment. (**E**) An asymmetrical anterior open bite is often associated with a digit sucking habit.

Local factors

Dento-alveolar, or local, factors have a more **localised effect** on the occlusion in comparison with skeletal and soft tissue factors. These factors are as follows.

Variations in tooth number

Hypodontia is a common condition characterised by developmental absence of one or more primary or secondary teeth excluding the third molars. In Caucasians, the most commonly missing teeth are: lower second premolar > upper lateral incisor > upper second premolar > lower central incisor. The aetiology of hypodontia is multifactorial with both inherited and environmental factors contributing to the condition. See Chapter 33 for further information.

Supernumerary teeth, defined as teeth in excess of the normal series, are most commonly found in the anterior maxillary region. Many different types exist including conical and tuberculate forms, supplemental teeth and odontomes. See Chapter 34 for further information.

The **early loss of deciduous teeth**, due to caries, trauma or root resorption, is a common occurrence. The effect this has on the developing dentition depends on the amount of crowding, the age of the patient and the tooth lost. In the presence of **crowding**, early tooth loss leads to space loss by drifting of adjacent teeth. When the dental arches are spaced, the loss of a deciduous tooth may have no impact on the developing permanent dentition. Concerning **age**, the younger the patient at the time of tooth loss, the greater the space loss likely to occur. Table 9.1 outlines the effect of the **tooth lost** on the developing dentition.

The most common **permanent tooth** to be extracted early is the **first permanent molar**. The occlusal consequences depend on which arch the tooth is lost from, the age at the time of loss and the degree of crowding. See Chapter 29 for further information.

A **permanent maxillary central incisor** can occasionally be lost due to trauma. If there is crowding, space loss can occur which may complicate later tooth replacement. In such cases, space maintenance with a removable appliance should be considered. This approach also has the advantage of replacement of a missing anterior tooth with its psychological benefits.

The effects of early loss of **premolars** depend on the degree of crowding, the age of the patient, the occlusion and the angulation of teeth adjacent to the extraction site. With increasing maturity and advanced root development, more tipping of adjacent teeth is likely to occur following extraction. However, if occlusal intercuspation is good, no movement may occur. If a first premolar is extracted and the adjacent canine is mesially angulated, the canine will upright favourably under lip pressure. If the canine is distally angulated it is unlikely to move.

Variation in tooth size

Tooth size is predominantly genetically determined. Teeth that are larger or smaller than normal are termed **macrodont** or **microdont**, respectively. Both macrodontia and microdontia may be generalised or localised. There is evidence that microdontia is associated with hypodontia whereas macrodontia is associated with the presence of supernumerary teeth. Macrodontia predisposes to dental crowding and microdontia predisposes to spacing. There is also evidence to suggest that microdontia of the maxillary lateral incisor is associated with impaction of the permanent maxillary canine. **Dento-alveolar disproportion** is the term given to the relative mismatch in tooth and jaw size that results in crowding or spacing.

The relative sum of the mesiodistal widths of the lower dentition compared with the upper determines how well the teeth interdigitate in occlusion. A mismatch in tooth size, termed a **Bolton discrepancy**, can be a limiting factor in achieving an ideal occlusal result.

Variation in tooth position

Infraocclusion occurs as a consequence of failure of eruption of a tooth due to **ankylosis** (the anatomical fusion of cementum and alveolar bone). As vertical skeletal development continues and the surrounding teeth erupt to compensate, an ankylosed tooth progressively submerges relative to its neighbours. Genetic factors have been implicated in ankylosis as siblings of affected patients often have this anomaly. The prevalence of infraocclusion has been reported to be between 1% and 9% with the first and second deciduous molars being most commonly affected. The prevalence of infraocclusion appears to be higher in those with hypodontia suggesting a common aetiological mechanism. Table 9.2 lists complications associated with infraocclusion. Complications such as tipping, inhibition of vertical development of adjacent teeth and deviation of the dental centreline to the affected side are the result of stretching of the transseptal periodontal fibres that interconnect the teeth (Figure 9.1A). The management of infraocclusion is summarised in Chapter 28.

Abnormalities in the position of teeth can also arise as a result of **tooth impaction**. Excluding third molars, commonly impacted teeth include maxillary canines, maxillary central incisors and first permanent molars. See Chapters 31 and 32 for further information.

Transposition is an abnormality where the position of teeth is interchanged. The maxillary canines and first premolars are the most commonly transposed teeth (Figure 9.1B). Genetic factors have been implicated in the aetiology of transposition.

Primary failure of eruption is a poorly understood condition, with a strong genetic basis, where a tooth fails to fully erupt (Figure 9.1C). The first and second permanent molars are most commonly affected. The eruptive mechanism may fail from commencement of root formation or once roots are partially developed and the tooth has undergone some eruptive movement. Teeth affected by this condition do not respond to orthodontic forces.

Frenal attachments

A low frenal attachment may be associated with a maxillary midline diastema (Figure 9.1Di). If the palatal papilla blanches on pulling the frenum and/or radiographically there is a alveolar cleft between the incisors (Figure 9.1Dii, iii), the frenum maybe implicated in diastema formation. In such cases, a frenectomy may be advisable as well as long-term retention of the corrected diastema. Rarely, a prominent lower labial frenum may persist that can cause problems with maintaining oral hygiene and be associated with a diastema (Figure 9.1Div). Recession may occur if the frenal attachment is to the gingival margin.

Habits

A prolonged **digit sucking** habit is one that exists until at least the age of 6–7 years when the permanent incisors have erupted. This can have a significant effect on the occlusion depending on the **duration** and **intensity** of the habit. When forces act on the teeth for **>6 hours a day**, tooth movement is likely to result. Occlusal effects include formation of an asymmetrical anterior open bite (Figure 9.1E), increased overjet and a unilateral buccal crossbite (see Chapter 30).

Table 10.1 The Angle classification of malocclusion.

Classification	Notes
Class I	The buccal groove of the mandibular first permanent molar should occlude with the mesio-buccal cusp of the maxillary first molar. This is considered to be the normal relationship.
Class II	The buccal groove of the mandibular first permanent molar occludes posterior to the mesio-buccal cusp of the maxillary first molar. The degree of discepancy is described as a fraction of the mesio-distal width of a premolar unit.
Division 1	The maxillary central incisors are proclined or normally inclined and the overjet is increased.
Division 2	The maxillary central incisors are retroclined.
Class III	The buccal groove of the mandibular first permanent molar occludes anterior to the mesio-buccal cusp of the maxillary first molar.

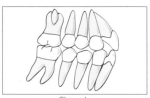
Class I

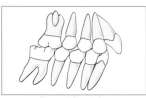
Class II (1/2 unit)

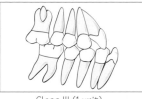
Class II (1 unit)

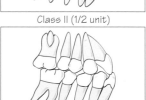
Class III (1/2 unit)

Class III (1 unit)

Table 10.2 The British Standards Institute's classification of incisor relationship.

Incisor classification	Definition
Class I	The lower incisor edges occlude on or lie below the cingulum plateau of the upper incisiors.
Class II, division 1	The lower incisor edges occlude behind the cingulum plateau of the upper incisors and the upper incisors are normally inclined or proclined.
Class II, division 2	The lower incisor edges occlude behind the cingulum plateau of the upper incisors and the upper incisors are retroclined.
Class III	The lower incisor edges occlude anterior to the cingulum plateau of the upper incisors.

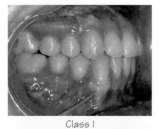
Class I

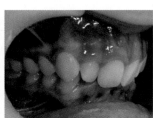
Class II, division 1

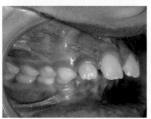
Class II, division 2

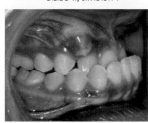
Class III

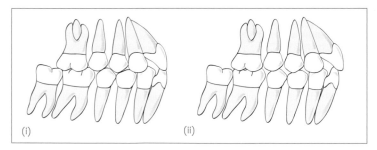

(i) (ii)

Figure 10.1 Andrews Class I molar relationship (i) results in better buccal intercuspation (note the maxillary premolar occlusion) than an Angle Class I relationship (ii) where the first molar is slightly further anteriorly positioned.

There are several classifications and indices of malocclusion. Some of these that are relevant to orthodontics are summarised below.

The Angle classification

The Angle classification of malocclusion was described by Edward H Angle in 1899 and is based on the relative anteroposterior (AP) position of the first permanent molars. Table 10.1 summarises this classification. Angle assumed that the first molars erupted in a constant position within the arches so that their relationship could be used to classify the AP skeletal relationship. This assumption is incorrect as the molar position can be influenced by other factors such as early loss of deciduous teeth (Chapter 9). If the position of the first molars has been influenced by such factors, or the teeth are missing, the incisor, premolar and/or canine relationship can be used to define the malocclusion.

Another disadvantage of the Angle classification is that the description of a Class I molar relationship has been outdated by **Andrews'** definition, which was based on the examination of a group of patients with ideal occlusion. Andrews found that the distobuccal cusp of the upper first permanent molar had to occlude with the mesiobuccal cusp of the lower second permanent molar for ideal buccal interdigitation. Figure 10.1 shows the difference between the Angle and Andrews Class I molar relationship.

Incisor classification

A classification of malocclusion based on the incisors is advantageous as treatment is often primarily aimed at correcting this relationship. The British Standards Institute incisor classification is summarised in Table 10.2. In clinical practice this is often used in association with the Angle molar classification.

Canine relationship

The canine relationship can be used as another method of classifying the AP occlusal relationship. The classification is outlined below:
• Class I – the maxillary permanent canine occludes in the embrasure between the lower canine and first premolar
• Class II – the maxillary canine occludes anterior to the embrasure between the lower canine and first premolar. The severity of the malrelationship can be described as a fraction of a tooth unit.
• Class III – the maxillary canine occludes posterior to the embrasure between the lower canine and first premolar

Index of Orthodontic Treatment Need (IOTN)

The IOTN was developed to help reduce the subjectivity in the assessment of treatment need. It ranks malocclusion in terms of the significance of various occlusal traits on an individual's dental health and perceived aesthetic impairment. There are two components of the index:
• Dental Health Component;
• Aesthetic Component.

Dental Health Component (DHC)

The DHC records the worst occlusal feature of the malocclusion that impacts on dental health. A **hierarchal scale** is used to identify the worst feature. In order of reducing dental health impact these are: **M**issing teeth > **O**verjet > **C**rossbite > **D**isplacement of contact points > **O**verbite. The acronym MOCDO can be used to remember this hierarchal scale. Once the worst occlusal feature has been recorded, the malocclusion can be characterised into one of five grades:
• Grade 1 – no need for treatment;
• Grade 2 – little need for treatment;
• Grade 3 – borderline need for treatment;
• Grade 4 and 5 – need for treatment.

See Appendix 1 for categorising the various occlusal features into the five grades.

Aesthetic Component

The Aesthetic Component consists of 10 colour photographs showing different levels of dental attractiveness (Appendix 1), which can be used to rate the attractiveness of individual cases. The patient is asked to choose a photograph which most closely represents their own dental appearance to give a score. Treatment need can be categorised according to the score given as follows:
• 1, 2 – no treatment need;
• 3,4 – small treatment need;
• 5–7 – moderate treatment need;
• 8–10 – definite treatment need.

A total score combining the DHC and Aesthetic Component can be given to define treatment need.

Peer Assessment Rating (PAR)

The PAR index has been developed as a tool for measuring malocclusion and assessing the quality of treatment results. Pre- and post-treatment study models are scored according to an assessment of various occlusal traits. The occlusal traits assessed include:
• Anterior crowding (×1) – upper and lower labial segment contact point displacements;
• Buccal occlusion (×1) – molar relationship, crossbites and lateral open bites;
• Overjet (×6);
• Overbite (×2);
• Centrelines (×4).

The score for each of these traits is multiplied by weighting factors (given in brackets above) that acknowledge that some occlusal traits bear more importance than others. A final score of 0 indicates perfect alignment and occlusion whilst higher scores indicate increasing levels of imperfection. The pre- and post-treatment scores can be compared to give a percentage improvement.

Principles of orthodontic treatment planning

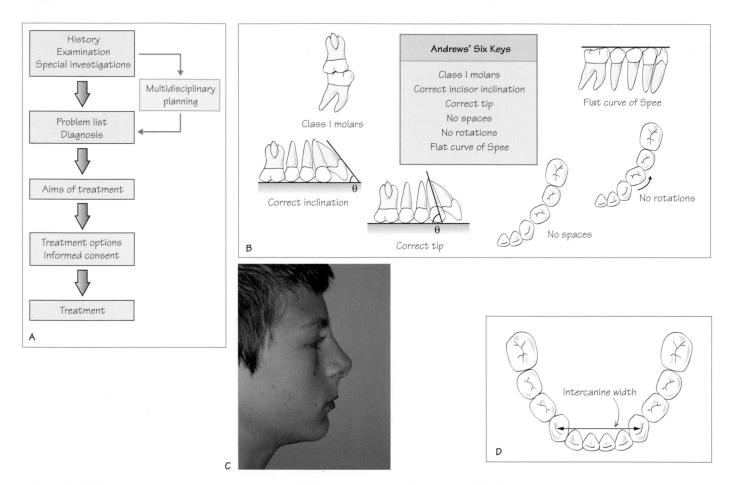

Figure 11.1 (**A**) The stages in orthodontic treatment planning. (**B**) Andrews' six keys for ideal occlusion. (**C**) This patient has an increased nasolabial angle and Class II division 1 malocclusion. It may be preferable to accept an increased overjet to limit upper incisor retraction and further loss of upper lip support. (**D**) The lower intercanine distance should be maintained during treatment to improve stability.

Table 11.1 Factors to be considered in the extraction *versus* non-extraction decision.

Factor	Comments
Medical history	It may be preferable to avoid extractions in patients with bleeding disorders
Patient preference	If a patient refuses extractions, consider other methods of space creation (e.g. headgear)
Compliance	Extractions maybe the only alternative if compliance with headgear is poor
Facial profile	Non-extraction treatment may be preferable if the lips are retrusive and the nasolabial angle is increased. Extraction treatment is preferable if the lips are too protrusive
Skeletal pattern	Space closure is more difficult if the vertical dimension is reduced. Extractions may be preferable if the vertical dimension is increased as they may prevent the overbite from reducing further
Unfavourable growth	The prospect of unfavourable growth during treatment may tip the balance towards mandibular extractions for incisor retraction in Class III cases if treatment is to be undertaken by orthodontics alone
Space required	A space analysis allows determination of space requirements
Dental health	Extraction should be considered if there are teeth with poor long-term prognosis (e.g. first permanent molars).
Tooth size discrepancies	Extracion treatment can help resolve tooth size discrepancies to improve occlusal fit (e.g. extraction of a lower incisor when the upper lateral incisors are microdont)

Orthodontic treatment planning includes history taking, clinical examination and consideration of special investigations. Following this it is possible to formulate a problem list and make a diagnosis, taking into consideration aetiological factors, and establish a list of treatment aims and provide a number of treatment options (Figure 11.1A). Important treatment planning considerations are discussed below.

Risk/cost–benefit analysis

Before commencing treatment it is essential to undertake a risk/cost–benefit analysis. See Chapter 12 for an in-depth discussion of factors that require consideration. It is important that the patient is motivated, dental disease is stabilised, oral hygiene is excellent and any habits such as digit sucking have ceased before placing appliances. **Informed consent**, with full discussion of the advantages and disadvantages of each treatment option, should be obtained and fully documented.

Addressing the patients concerns

For patient satisfaction at the end of treatment, it is important to address the patient's concerns within the treatment plan. It is beneficial to spend time during history taking to explore these in detail. If the patient's concerns cannot be addressed it is essential that these are discussed as part of the informed consent process.

Multidisciplinary treatment planning

A large number of patients require complex treatment that crosses the boundary between specialities. Many orthodontic patients fall into this category (e.g. hypodontia, orthognathic surgery). For best results, treatment should be planned following a meeting between all clinicians involved in the patient's care. If the general dentist is not directly involved in providing treatment, they should be informed of the treatment plan.

Aims of treatment

It is important before commencing treatment to have clear aims and objectives. **Andrews** described six **keys** (Figure 11.1B) that are important in achieving an ideal occlusion. This may not always be possible in patients with skeletal discrepancies, in whom the incisors are not normally inclined or vertically positioned, and in those with tooth size discrepancies (Bolton discrepancy, see Chapter 9). If premolar teeth are extracted in one arch and not in the other, it is not possible to achieve a Class I molar relationship, although this is not essential.

It is not possible to treat all patients to an ideal occlusion. For example, a patient with a severe skeletal discrepancy may not be willing to undergo orthognathic surgery, and the treatment aim may be limited to alignment only whilst accepting the inter-arch relationship. Another example occasionally encountered is a patient with Class II malocclusion, retrusive lips and an obtuse nasolabial angle (Figure 11.1C). In such a case, it may be preferable to accept an overjet, and not fully retract the upper incisors, in order to maintain upper lip support and prevent further lip retrusion.

Treatment timing

Although orthodontics can be undertaken at any age, the majority of treatment is carried out during the early permanent dentition stage with a number of advantages:

- most teeth are present and can be incorporated into the fixed appliances;
- compliance may be better in the early rather than later teens;
- growth can facilitate space closure, overbite and overjet reduction;
- advantage can be taken of the leeway space for alignment.

Interceptive treatment (Chapter 28) may be undertaken earlier if it benefits dental health (e.g. crossbite correction), facilitates later treatment (e.g. balancing/compensating extractions) or has psychological advantages (e.g. overjet reduction). Joint orthodontic-orthognathic treatment is usually done later so that surgery coincides with the cessation of facial growth which is approximately 19 years in males and 17 years in females.

Importance of the lower incisor position

The lower incisors erupt into a position of muscular balance between the lips and the tongue. An aim of treatment is often to maintain the lower incisor anteroposterior position to maximise post-treatment stability. If the lower incisors are proclined during treatment they are likely to upright under lip pressure following appliance removal with re-emergence of crowding unless permanently retained. There are some exceptions to this rule where it may be acceptable to alter the lower incisor position, such as:

- if a lip trap, that will be corrected following treatment, has resulted in lower incisor retroclination;
- in a digit sucker in whom the habit has artificially retroclined the incisors;
- in Class II malocclusion (e.g. Class II division 2) where a deep overbite has resulted in posterior incisor trapping;
- in Class III malocclusion where there is sufficient overbite to maintain a retracted lower incisor position;
- in cases requiring orthognathic surgery where a new position of soft tissue balance will be established following surgery.

As well as lower incisor position, it is generally important to maintain the lower **intercanine distance** (Figure 11.1D) as evidence suggests that an increase is highly unstable unless the canines are lingually placed before treatment commences.

Because the dimensions of the lower arch often have to be accepted, the position of the upper arch is dictated by and planned around the lower arch.

Extraction versus non-extraction

A number of factors need to be considered when determining whether to adopt an extraction or non-extraction approach during treatment (Table 11.1). Methods available for space creation are summarised in Chapter 18. All comprehensive orthodontic treatment should involve a formal space analysis (Chapter 18) to plan **anchorage** requirements.

Limitations of orthodontic treatment

The skeletal pattern and facial growth can be major limiting factors in orthodontics. With favourable growth, it is possible to correct a mild skeletal discrepancy by **dentoalveolar compensation** to **camouflage** the underlying discrepancy with fixed or functional appliances. When the skeletal discrepancy is more severe, this approach may not be appropriate and surgical correction may be required.

Type of appliance used

Removable appliances (see Chapter 38) are suitable for simple tipping movement, to aid overbite reduction and for expansion. Fixed appliances (see Chapter 40) can achieve bodily tooth movement and are beneficial when three-dimensional control with multiple tooth movements is required.

Retention

Retention is the process of retaining corrected tooth positions (see Chapter 41). The majority of patients benefit from long-term wear of retainers to prevent relapse and **late lower incisor crowding**. Spacing, rotations and changes in lower incisor position are particularly prone to relapse. Fixed retention can be considered in such cases.

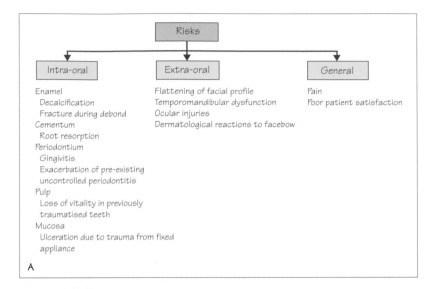

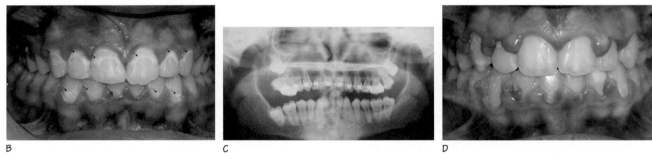

Figure 12.1 (**A**) The risks of orthodontic treatment. (**B**) Enamel decalcification associated with orthodontic treatment. This commonly occurs located adjacent to the gingival margin where plaque readily accumulates. (**C**) A rare example of severe root resorption following fixed appliance therapy: it can be seen that the maxillary incisor roots are resorbed. (**D**) Gingival hyperplasia during orthodontic treatment.

The decision to undergo orthodontic treatment should be based upon an evaluation of the risks and benefits of the procedure (**risk–benefit analysis**). The aim of this chapter is to give an overview of the factors that require consideration during the treatment planning stage.

Benefits of orthodontic treatment
The benefits of orthodontic treatment can be considered under the following headings:
• Psychological;
• Dental health;
• Functional.

Psychological benefits
The smile is an important component of an attractive facial appearance. Malocclusion may affect **self-esteem** and **social interaction**, and can be a focus of **teasing**. Individuals with similar degrees of malocclusion can be affected differently depending on their self-esteem. Therefore, it should not always be assumed that any given dental irregularity will require treatment from the point of psychological benefits. There is evid-

ence to suggest that orthodontic treatment can lead to an improvement in self-esteem and psychological health in those whose malocclusion is affecting them psychologically.

Dental health benefits
Dental health benefits of orthodontic treatment include:
• A reduction in the risk of sustaining **traumatic dental injuries**. An increased overjet and lip incompetence increases the susceptibility of the upper incisors to traumatic dental injuries. The risk of traumatic injury is proportional to the size of the overjet as shown in Table 12.1.

Table 12.1	
Overjet	**Prevalence of incisor trauma**
5 mm	22%
9 mm	24%
>9 mm	44%

• A reduction in complications associated with **mandibular displacement**. A posterior crossbite associated with a lateral mandibular displacement *may* predispose to temporomandibular joint dysfunction within a susceptible patient. An anterior crossbite associated with a mandibular displacement can exacerbate toothwear of the incisal edges and compromise the periodontal health of the lower incisors.

• A reduction in complications associated with **deep traumatic overbite**. A traumatic overbite may aggravate periodontal destruction of the upper palatal and lower labial gingivae if oral hygiene is poor. A deep overbite can also potentiate toothwear at the site where the incisors shear past each other.

• A reduction in complications associated with **impacted teeth**. Impacted teeth may resorb the roots of adjacent teeth and their dental follicle may undergo cystic change in rare circumstances.

• A reduction in **caries** and improvement of **periodontal health**? There is no evidence that the correction of malocclusion leads to later reduction in caries and periodontal disease. Dietary factors, oral hygiene and host susceptibility are more important in determining disease initiation and progression. Patients with crowding can often still maintain good oral hygiene by adapting their tooth brushing technique.

Functional benefits

Functional benefits of orthodontic treatment may include:

• An improvement in **masticatory efficiency**. The ability to incise and chew food can be compromised by anterior and posterior open bites, severe hypodontia and severe Class III malocclusion. Most patients develop compensatory mechanisms for this reduced efficiency. Although nutritionally there may be minimal impact, a patient may find it embarrassing to eat in public places if it is difficult to incise food normally.

• An improvement of **temporomandibular joint dysfunction** (TMD)? There is no evidence that orthodontic treatment can lead to long-term improvement of TMD.

• An improvement in **speech**? There is very little evidence to suggest that orthodontic treatment can lead to an improvement in speech in those with speech defects.

The risks of orthodontic treatment

The potential risks of orthodontic treatment are outlined in Figure 12.1A.

Decalcification is a common occurrence following orthodontic treatment. Plaque accumulates around orthodontic brackets and underneath archwires to initiate caries if the diet is cariogenic. This may present as white/brown areas of decalcification (Figure 12.1B) or cavitation in severe cases. Any tooth can be affected but when the anterior labial surfaces are involved, this has the greatest aesthetic impact. Decalcification can be prevented by rigorous oral hygiene control, dietary advice and use of topical fluoride supplements.

Small amounts (1–2 mm) of **root resorption**, with little long-term implications, occurs in the majority of patients undergoing fixed appliance treatment. Approximately 15% of patients maybe affected by >2.5 mm loss of root length (Figure 12.1C), which may have long-term implications especially if superimposed on periodontal bone loss. Root resorption is thought to occur as a consequence of orthodontic forces exceeding capillary pressure and producing areas of necrosis. The necrotic tissue is cleared away by multinucleated giant cells which also remove exposed cementum and dentine in severe cases (see Chapter 35). Risk factors for orthodontic-related root resorption are summarised in Box 12.1.

Many patients will experience **gingivitis** and **gingival hyperplasia** during fixed appliance treatment if oral hygiene is not optimal (Figure 12.1D). This usually resolves following appliance removal with no long-term complications. If orthodontic treatment is undertaken in uncontrolled **periodontal disease**, there is a higher risk of alveolar bone loss and gingival recession.

There is a small risk of **loss of vitality** in teeth that have previously suffered trauma during orthodontic treatment. Traumatic injuries can produce degenerative changes within the pulp that reduce its ability to cope with orthodontic tooth movement.

There has been much debate about whether orthodontic treatment involving extractions can lead to flattening of the **facial profile** as a result of incisor retraction. The evidence would suggest that extraction therapy has a minimal effect on the facial profile in the average patient. However, care should be taken in those with already retrusive lips and an obtuse nasolabial angle when planning extractions for incisor retraction (Figure 11.1C).

Orthodontic treatment has been implicated in the aetiology of **temporomandibular joint dysfunction**. The evidence for a causal link is very weak.

There have been reported cases of **ocular injury**, leading to blindness, due to trauma from the facebow component of headgear. Injuries can occur if the facebow disengages its intra-oral attachment during sleep or if it is pulled out by another child. This can result in the facebow catapulting back into the face with potential to damage the eyes. It is essential that all headgears used have appropriate safety devices to prevent such injuries (see Chapter 37).

In patients sensitive to nickel, contact between the facebow and skin can trigger an **allergic response**. Either a plastic coated facebow, or one covered in adhesive tape, should be used to prevent such reactions in susceptible patients. Intra-oral reactions to nickel are extremely rare even in patients displaying dermatological reactions.

Pain is commonly encountered by patients during orthodontic tooth movement (see Chapter 40). This may be caused by the inflammatory response that accompanies tooth movement (see Chapter 35) or by mucosal ulceration as a result of trauma from appliance components. The intensity of the pain can show large individual variation and it is important to warn all patients about its possibility before commencing treatment.

Poor patient satisfaction following treatment is disappointing for both the patient and clinician undertaking treatment. This can arise if the primary concerns of the patient have not been addressed, in the event of unexplained complications and following **relapse**. Fully informed patients are less likely to be dissatisfied at the end of treatment even in the event of minor complications. The necessity for retention should be carefully discussed and documented in all cases during treatment planning.

Table 13.1 The orthodontic significance of some medical conditions.

Medical condition	Orthodontic significance
Bleeding disorders (e.g. von Willibrand's disease, haemophilia, renal disease)	• Avoid extraction treatment if possible • Minimise risk of mucosal injury from fixed appliances, e.g. avoid steel ligatures/ties, use low-profile brackets, turn down archwire ends
Epilepsy	• Ensure epilepsy is well controlled before commencing treatment • Risk of dental/mucosal injury or aspiration of broken appliances during fits
Latex allergy	• Confirm allergy with doctor • Treat at beginning of day to minimise exposure to environmental latex • Use latex-free gloves, elastomeric modules and elastics
Nickel allergy	• Confirm allergy with doctor • Oral mucosal reactions are rare even in sensitised individuals • Safe to use stainless steel within mouth as little nickel release • Use plastic-coated headgear to avoid skin reaction • Avoid nickel-titanium archwires. Alternative materials: stainless steel, titanium-molybdenum alloy and gold

Table 13.2 Orthodontic management of patients at high, moderate and low risk of infective endocarditis.

	Before orthodontics	During orthodontics (once level of risk confirmed)
High risk	• Consult cardiologist • Ensure good dental health • Ensure good oral hygiene (OH)	• Avoid gingival trauma • Use bonded attachments on molars if possible (i.e. avoid bands and separators). • Chlorhexidine (0.2%) rinse before adjustments • Antibiotic cover for banding, debanding, separators, extractions, scaling and polishing • Regularly reinforce OH
Moderate risk	As above	As above
Low risk	As above	No special precautions

Table 13.4 Syndromes with oro-facial features impacting on orthodontic treatment.

Syndrome	Orthodonic features	Medical features
Down syndrome	Maxillary hypoplasia, Class III, anterior openbite (AOB), crossbites, hypodontia, microdontia, periodontal disease, macroglossia and cleft lip and palate	Learning disability, congenital heart defects, epilepsy, atlanto-axial immobility, immunodeficiency
Ectodermal dysplasia	Anodontia/hypodontia, microdontia, xerostomia and Class III malocclusion	Hypohidrosis (↓ sweating) and hypotrichosis (↓ hair).
Cleidocranial dysplasia	Multiple supernumeraries, persistence of deciduous teeth, multiple unerupted teeth, dentigerous cysts, maxillary hypoplasia and Class III Malocclusion	Clavicles defective or absent, frontal bossing and depressed nasal bridge
Craniosynostosis (e.g. Crouzon/Apert's syndrome)	Maxillary hypoplasia and Class III malocclusion	Increased intracranial pressure, sleep apnoea, ocular proptosis and hearing defects
Muscular dystrophy	Increased face height and AOB	Progressive muscle weakness, cardiomyopathies, respiratory disease, malignant hyperthermia

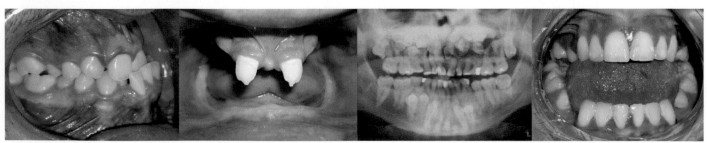

Down syndrome	Ectodermal dysplasia	Cleidocranial dysplasia	Muscular dystrophy
Class III malocclusion	Severe hypodontia	Multiple supernumeraries	Anterior open bite

History taking is an essential component of diagnosis and treatment planning. This chapter outlines the main components of the history that are relevant to orthodontic practice.

The patient's concerns

For **patient satisfaction** following treatment, it is important to address the patient's main reason(s) for seeking care. Patients seek orthodontic treatment for a number of reasons (Box 13.1), of which improvement in aesthetics is the most common. It is important to list the main improvements the patient wishes to achieve, in order of importance, and address these during treatment planning. If it is not possible to fully address the patient's concerns, for example due to anatomical limitations, this should be explained as part of informed consent. If the patient is a child, their views should be sought first before seeking the opinion of their parents.

Box 13.1 Reasons for seeking orthodontic treatment

- Improvement in dental aesthetics
- Improvement in facial aesthetics
- Dentist's advice
- Problems eating, in particular, incising food
- Traumatic overbite
- Facilitation of restorative treatment
- Improved access for tooth brushing
- Speech problems
- Sleep apnoea

It is also important to gauge the patient's **motivation** for treatment at this stage. Motivation may be:

- **internal** – where the desire to seek treatment comes from within;
- **external** – where the desire for treatment is influenced by others, e.g. pressure from a parent.

External motivation is more likely to lead to problems with compliance, such as maintaining adequate oral hygiene, and less patient satisfaction at the end of treatment. It is usually clear when motivation is external as the parent may try to dominate the discussion by speaking on behalf of the patient. The patient's enthusiasm to undergo fixed appliance treatment, which may involve extractions, is often a good indicator of motivation for treatment.

Dental history

The dental history can also give valuable information about motivation regarding dental health. Poor oral hygiene routines, irregular past dental attendance and the presence of numerous carious cavities or restorations can indicate potential problems with compliance. It is important not to always assume this as some patients may have undergone extensive treatment during childhood and since then changed their attitude towards dental health. Patients should be registered with a general dentist and have regular dental check-ups during orthodontic treatment.

Other important aspects that should be explored in the history are:

- digit sucking habits;
- dental trauma – traumatised teeth may be more prone to orthodontically induced root resorption and may be at greater risk of becoming non-vital with tooth movement;

- nail biting/pen chewing habits – these can potentiate orthodontically induced root resorption;
- bruxism.

Finally, it is important to establish if there has been previous orthodontic treatment and if so the duration, type of appliance(s) used, extractions involved and any problems faced during care. In such cases, it can be beneficial to request records from the previous orthodontist to gain details about the original malocclusion.

Family and social history

It is often useful to find out if other members of the family have experience of orthodontic treatment. If so, the patient is more likely to understand the commitment required for successful treatment.

The family history can also be relevant at times as some dental traits have a genetic component. For example, hypodontia and mandibular prognathism can run in families. The degree of mandibular prognathism in other family members may give an indication of the likely pattern of future mandibular growth.

Finally, as will all patients, it is important to ask about habits such as smoking and alcohol consumption as these can affect oral health.

Medical history

A number of medical conditions can influence how orthodontic treatment is delivered. Because more children are surviving illnesses that were previously fatal and more treatment is being undertaken in adults, it is becoming commoner to encounter patients with complex medical histories. Some conditions, particularly syndromes, can also influence the pattern of craniofacial development.

Table 13.1 lists some common medical conditions that may influence orthodontic treatment and Table 13.2 outlines the orthodontic management of patients at risk of infective endocarditis. Table 13.3 lists medications that may alter the rate of orthodontic tooth movement if used for chronic conditions. Table 13.4 lists some syndromes that may manifest with orthodontic problems.

Table 13.3 The effect of long-term use of some popular medications on bone metabolism and tooth movement.

	Effect on bone metabolism	Effect on tooth movement
Non-steroidal anti-inflammatory drugs		
Aspirin	↓	↓
Ibuprofen	↓	↓
Diclofenac	↓	↓
Corticosteroids	↑	↑
Bisphosphonates	↓	↓
Paracetamol	?	No effect

As a general principle, it is important to liaise with the patient's doctor if there are any doubts about the medical history or concerns about how a medical condition may influence the delivery of dental care. The patient's doctor should also be consulted to determine the level of risk (i.e. high, medium and low) in those who maybe prone to bacterial endocarditis.

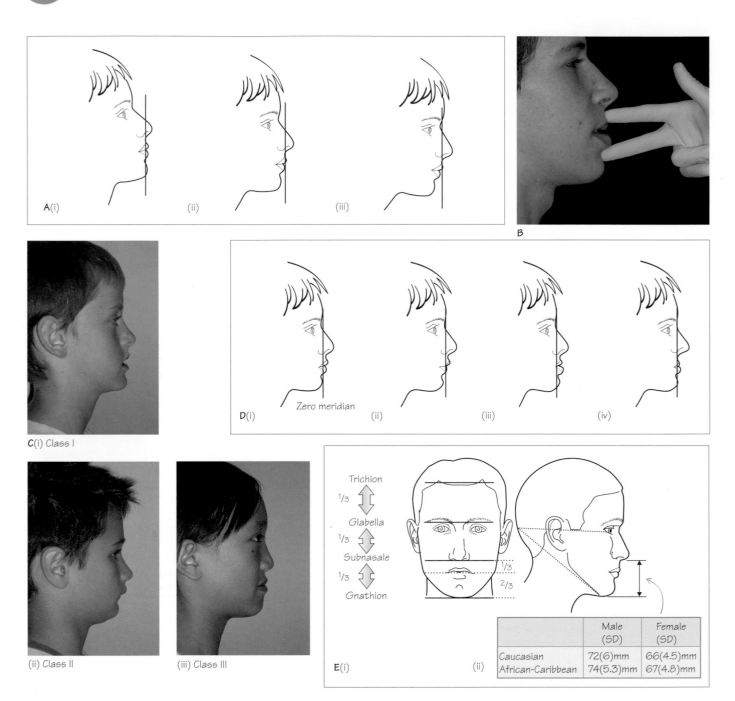

Figure 14.1 (**A**) The orientation of the head can affect the assessment of the AP skeletal pattern. Ideally, the head should be in the natural head position (ii) to achieve this, the patient should be sitting upright, relaxed, and looking straight ahead at a distant point at eye level. Incorrect head posture can lead to an inaccurate assessment of skeletal pattern (i, iii). (**B**) Assessment of the AP skeletal pattern. (**C**) An example of a (i) skeletal I, (ii) skeletal II and (iii) skeletal III pattern. (**D**) The zero meridian can be used to assess AP jaw position in relationship to the cranial base and gives an indication of which jaw(s) is contributing to the skeletal discrepancy. (i) Normally, the base of the upper lip should lie 2–3 mm ahead and the lower lip 0–2 mm behind this line. (ii) Class II pattern due to mandibular retrognathia. (iii) Class III pattern due to mandibular protrusion. (iv) Class III pattern due to maxillary retrusion. (**E**) Assessment of the vertical dimension by (i) examining the proportional relationship of the LAFH to the mid-face and (ii) assessment of the FMPA and absolute LAFH.

Orthodontic examination should begin as soon as the patient enters the surgery. The **general stage of development**, of which statural height is a good indicator, should be noted. The presence of secondary sexual characteristics (Figure 2.1D) also provides a good indication of developmental stage. This chapter will focus on the assessment of skeletal pattern.

Assessment of skeletal pattern

The relative position of the maxilla and mandible, termed the skeletal pattern, has a large influence on the relationship of the maxillary and mandibular dentitions. The skeletal pattern should be assessed in three dimensions:
- Anteroposterior (AP);
- Vertical;
- Transverse.

Anteroposterior dimension

The aim is to relate the AP position of the mandible to the maxilla and the relationship of these bones to the cranial base. Assessment of the position of each jaw relative to the cranial base gives an indication of which jaw has contributed to any discrepancy. It is important to assess the patient in the **natural head position**, which is a standardised reproducible head orientation, as the tilt of the head can influence the interpretation of skeletal pattern (Figure 14.1A). To achieve this, the patient should be sitting upright, relaxed, and looking straight ahead at a distant point at eye level and the teeth should be lightly in occlusion.

The most anterior part of the maxilla and the mandible can be palpated in the midline through the base of the lips (Figure 14.1B). The relationship of the mandible relative to the maxilla can be classified as follows:
- **Class I** – when the mandible lies 2–3 mm posterior to the maxilla. The profile is straight (Figure 14.1Ci).
- **Class II** – when the mandible is retrusive relative to the maxilla. The profile is convex. The discrepancy should be termed mild, moderate or severe (Figure 14.Cii).
- **Class III** – when the maxilla is retrusive relative to the mandible. The profile is concave. The discrepancy should be termed mild, moderate or severe (Figure 14.Ciii).

To determine the position of the jaws relative to the cranial base, imagine a vertical line drawn through soft tissue nasion in the natural head position (Figure 14.1Di). This line is termed the **zero meridian** and represents the anterior limit of the cranial base. In Caucasians the anterior limit of the base of the upper lip (soft tissue A-point) should lie 2–3 mm ahead and the base of the lower lip (soft tissue B-point) 0–2 mm behind the zero meridian. When making this assessment, it is important to remember that there is **ethnic variation** in normal lower face protrusion. The face progressively becomes less protrusive as follows: African Caribbeans > Asians > white people of northern European ancestry. The term used to indicate that both jaws are protrusive is **bimaxillary protrusion**, which is a common feature in African Caribbean people. Figure 14.1D shows some examples of various AP relationships. As well as using the zero meridian as a guide, other signs which *may* be present and are suggestive of maxillary retrusion include:
- paranasal flattening;
- an obtuse nasolabial angle;
- reduced incisor show at rest;
- prominent nasolabial folds;
- a flat nasal bridge;
- lower scleral show.

Vertical dimension

The vertical skeletal dimension can influence the degree of vertical incisor overlap, lip competency and overall facial aesthetics. There are two methods with which the vertical dimension should be assessed:
- lower anterior face height (LAFH) proportion;
- Frankfort–mandibular planes angle (FMPA).

Vertically in the frontal view, the face can be split into thirds (Figure 14.1E). The LAFH (subnasale–gnathion) should be approximately equal to the middle face height (glabella–subnasale) for facial balance. However, if the middle face height is incorrect, the LAFH may be proportional to it but also incorrect such that incisor overlap and lip competency are adversely affected. This is why some clinicians also measure the **absolute LAFH**. The normal absolute measurements for LAFH are given in the table in Figure 14.1E.

The LAFH can also be split into thirds and ideally the upper lip should represent one-third of the total height (Figure 14.1E).

The FMPA is assessed in the profile view (Figure 14.1E) and also gives an indication of the vertical dimension. It measures the relationship between the LAFH and posterior face height (i.e. ramus height). It is considered to be normal when the lines representing the mandibular and Frankfort planes intersect in the occipital region. If the point of intersection is anterior to the occiput, the vertical dimension is usually increased and if it lies posterior to the occiput, it is reduced.

Transverse dimension

The two components of the transverse dimension that should be assessed are:
- facial symmetry;
- arch width.

It is quite common to find asymmetries in the face but those that affect the mandible and maxilla are particularly important when planning orthodontic treatment.

The **symmetry** of facial structures can be assessed by constructing a **facial midline** between soft tissue nasion and the middle part of the upper lip at the vermillion border. The chin point should be coincident with this line. If there is an asymmetry of the chin point, it is also important to check for a **compensatory cant** in the maxillary occlusal plane. Mild asymmetries in the chin point can be produced by a lateral **mandibular displacement** on closing if there is an occlusal interference. See Chapter 25 to read about asymmetries in more detail.

The relative width of the upper and lower arches affects the transverse relationship of the teeth. Often the maxilla is narrow which results in a crossbite of the buccal segments if there has been inadequate dentoalveolar compensation. On intra-oral palpation, the maxilla should be slightly wider than the mandible at corresponding points. It is important to remember that the absolute transverse dimensions of the maxilla may be normal, but a *relative* transverse maxillary discrepancy, manifesting as a posterior crossbite, may exist due to incorrect AP positioning of the maxilla/mandible (Figure 8.1C). The AP position can affect the transverse relationship as the dental arches get wider as one moves distally.

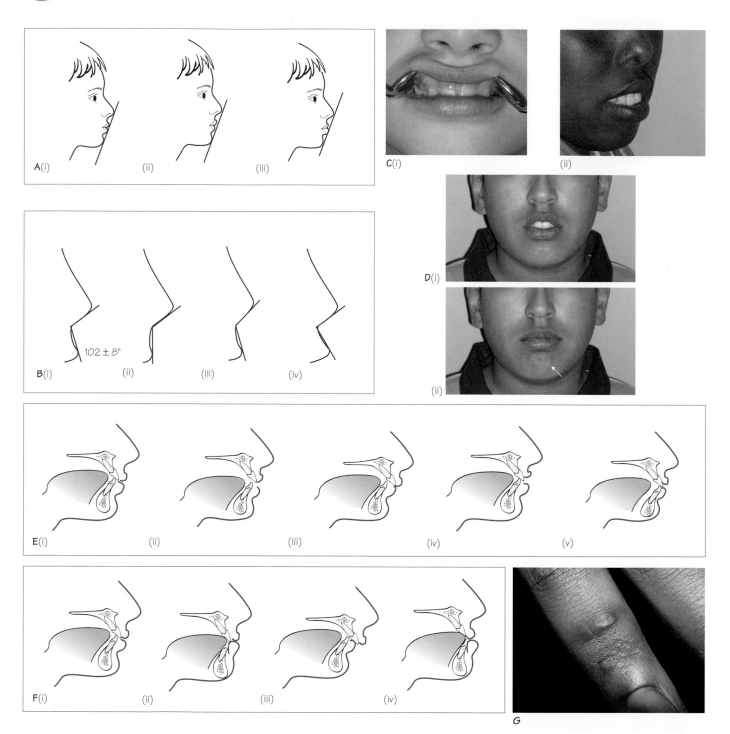

Figure 15.1 (**A**) Assessment of lower lip fullness in relationship to Ricketts E-line: (i) normal, (ii) retrusive and (iii) full lower lip. (**B**) The nasolabial angle may be (i) normal, (ii) obtuse due to a poor upper lip position, (iii) obtuse due to an upwardly sloping columella and normal upper lip position and (iv) acute due to a protrusive upper lip. (**C**) The lower lip line can influence incisor position. (i) A high lower lip line is associated with retroclined upper incisors and (ii) a low lower lip line is associated with incisor proclination and poor stability of overjet correction. (**D**) Excessive muscular activity to close the lips is indicated by puckering of the chin due to mentalis contraction. (**E**) A number of factors determine lip competency. (i) Competent lips. Incompetent lips due to (ii) an increased LAFH, (iii) mandibular retrognathia, (iv) a short upper lip and (v) incisor protrusion. (**F**) Methods of achieving an anterior oral seal: (i) lip to lip, (ii) tongue to lower lip, (iii) lower lip to palate and (iv) tongue to upper lip contact. (**G**) a vigorous digit sucking habit can leave a tell tale colour on the digit sucked where it rubs against the incisal edges.

As well as the skeletal pattern, the facial soft tissues can influence tooth position. If there is an underlying skeletal discrepancy, the soft tissues may help to guide teeth into a more favourable position (**dento-alveolar compensation**) so that the occlusal relationship is improved. Soft tissue evaluation should involve examination of:

The lips

The following aspects of the lips should be examined:
- lip fullness and nasolabial angle;
- lip tone;
- lower lip line;
- lip competency;
- method of achieving an anterior oral seal at rest/swallowing.

Lip fullness maybe classified as **protrusive**, **straight** or **retrusive**. The relationship of the lips to **Ricketts Esthetic line (E-line)**, which runs between the tip of the nose and chin point, can help with this assessment (Figure 15.1A). If the lower lip lies anterior to the line it is considered protrusive, if it lies 0–2 mm behind it is normal and if >2 mm posterior to the line it is retrusive. If the nose is large, so that the E-line is displaced anteriorly, this may give a misleading assessment. The lips tend to become less protrusive with growth as the nose and chin point develop (see Chapter 6).

The **nasolabial angle** (NLA), formed by a tangent to the upper lip and columella of the nose, can give an indication of upper lip position (Figure 15.1B). In Caucasians, the upper lip should slope slightly anteriorly (8–14°) to the vertical. The NLA can be classified as normal (102 ± 8° for males and females), acute (<90°) or obtuse (>90°). It may be increased, with a relatively normal upper lip position, if the columella of the nose slopes upwards excessively. There is **ethnic variation**, and it is normal for African Caribbeans to have an acute NLA.

The profile can influence the **extraction/non-extraction** decision (Table 11.1).

Regarding **tonicity**, the lips may be **flaccid**, which means there is little muscular tone, have normal tone or be **highly active**. The term **strap-like lower lip** is given to a highly active lower lip. Lip tonicity can influence the position of muscular balance such that incisors tend to be more protrusive with reducing tonicity. If the lips are very active the incisors may be retroclined.

The **lower lip line** is the vertical relationship between the lower lip and maxillary incisors at rest. It is determined by the lower anterior face height (LAFH), anteroposterior (AP) mandibular position and the lower lip length. Ideally, the lower lip should lie adjacent to the middle third of the maxillary central incisor crowns. In Class II division 1 malocclusion the lip line can be lower, leading to proclination of the upper incisors and in Class II division 2 malocclusion it can be high leading to their retroclination (Figure 15.1C). In Class II division 1 the stability of overjet correction is questionable if the lower lip does not cover at least the incisal third of the maxillary central incisors at rest.

The lips may be described as:
- **Competent** – a lip seal is produced with minimal muscular effort when the mandible is in the rest position.
- **Potentially competent** – the positioning of the upper incisors prevents a comfortable lip seal from being obtained.
- **Incompetent** – excessive muscular activity is required to produce a lip seal. Signs of excessive activity include puckering of the skin overlying the chin, due to mentalis contraction, and flattening of the labiomental fold when the lips are held together (Figure 15.1D). If the inter-labial distance at rest is >4 mm the lips can be considered

incompetent. Patients may learn to habitually keep the lips together with increased muscular effort and forward mandibular posturing.

Factors that influence lip competency (Figure 15.1E) include age (↑ age → ↓ lip separation; page 12), LAFH (↑ LAFH → ↑ lip separation), AP mandibular position (↑ mandibular retrognathia → ↑ lip separation), lip length (normal upper lip length in females = 20–22 mm, and in males = 22–24 mm) and upper incisor position (↑ protrusion → ↑ lip separation).

The significance of lip competence lies in the **stability** of Class II division 1 malocclusion correction. If the lips fail to control upper incisor position following treatment there is a significant risk of relapse.

An **anterior oral seal** at rest and during swallowing can be created by a number of mechanisms (Figure 15.1F):
- lip to lip contact (± mandibular forward posturing);
- tongue to lower lip contact;
- lower lip to palate contact;
- tongue to upper lip contact.

When a *lip to lip* seal can not be attained, an **adaptive swallowing pattern** must be produced to prevent expulsion of oral contents during swallowing. A *tongue to lower lip* seal (also termed an **adaptive tongue thrust**) is often found in Class II division 1 malocclusion and a clue to its existence is an overbite that is just incomplete. A *lower lip to palate* seal is also found with Class II division 1 malocclusions, when the lower lip is caught behind the upper incisors (**lower lip trap**, Figure 8.1E). This often results in proclination of the upper incisors and retroclination of the lower incisors. A *tongue to upper lip* seal is sometimes seen in Class III malocclusions.

Tongue

It is difficult to assess the **size** and **position** of the tongue unless it is grossly abnormal.

During **function**, there may be an **adaptive tongue thrust** where the tongue is positioned anteriorly to help achieve a lip seal when the lips are incompetent. This adaptive mechanism often disappears following occlusal correction. Rarely, a patient may present with an **endogenous tongue thrust** where the tongue is thrust forward forcibly during swallowing due to a neuromuscular defect. **Macroglossia** is rarely seen and is difficult to diagnose unless it is moderate/severe. Signs of a tongue thrust and macroglossia include:
- proclination of the upper and lower incisors;
- reverse curve of Spee in the lower arch;
- anterior open bite;
- presence of a lisp;
- tongue interposed between the incisors at rest;
- crenulation of the lateral border of the tongue.

Such findings should alert the clinician to the high risk of relapse if the AP incisor position is altered.

Habits

A clue to the presence of a vigorous **digit sucking** habit is the presence of a callous on the digit sucked in the area in contact with the incisors (Figure 15.1G). **Nail biting** habits can potentiate orthodontically induced root resorption and are easily identified by examining the nails.

TMJ

It is important to note the presence of tenderness of the muscles of mastication, the existence of clicking or crepitus and the range of mandibular movements during orthodontic assessment. If pathology is found, there may be a history of parafunction or facial trauma.

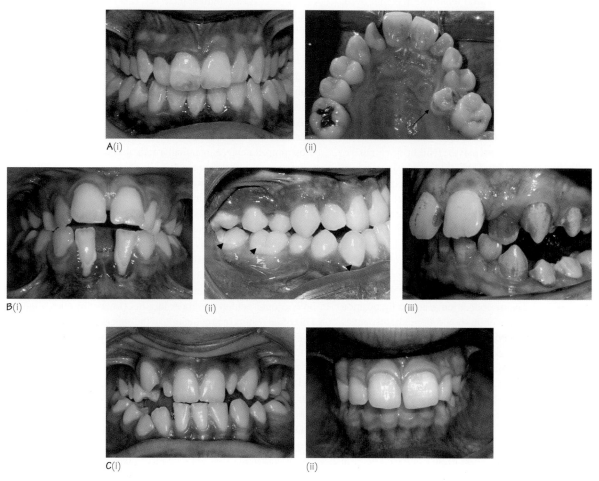

A(i)   (ii)

B(i)   (ii)   (iii)

C(i)   (ii)

Figure 16.1 (**A**) (i) Enamel hypomineralisation should be documented before commencing treatment. It can affect dental aesthetics and bond strength of orthodontic attachments. (ii) Often severely hypoplastic premolars make good candidates for extraction if space is required for dental alignment. (**B**) Indicators of poor oral hygiene: (i) gingival inflammation, recession and plaque deposits are clearly visible, (ii) lines of decalcification are seen following the gingival margin of the first molars and (iii) plaque demonstrated using disclosing tablets. (**C**) Developmental disturbances in tooth size: (i) microdontia of the maxillary lateral incisors and (ii) megadontia of the upper left central incisor.

The aims of intra-oral examination are to:
- assess the mucosal/dental surfaces for pathology;
- determine the level of oral hygiene;
- establish whether dental development is normal;
- assess tooth position within and between the arches.

Assessment for pathology

Every patient should have a full examination of the mucosal surfaces during routine assessment. Dental pathology can have a significant influence on treatment planning. Of particular relevance are:
- dental caries;
- dental hypoplasia and hypomineralisation;
- toothwear;
- sequelae of traumatic injuries to the dentition;
- gingivitis, periodontitis and gingival recession.

All teeth that have previously suffered trauma or have advanced caries or large restorations should undergo thermal or electrical **vitality testing**. Areas of significant enamel **hypoplasia/hypomineralisation** should be documented and photographed (Figure 16.1A). Patients often become more aware of these defects during treatment as their primary focus of attention, the dental irregularity, is corrected. This may lead them to incorrectly attributing the enamel defects to orthodontic treatment. **Periodontal charting** is important if periodontitis is suspected. All dental disease *must* be controlled before contemplating orthodontic treatment.

Oral hygiene

The level of oral hygiene can be assessed by examining for gingivitis, probing to elicit gingival bleeding, and with visual aids such as disclosing tablets/solution (Figure 16.1B). The presence of a line of decalcification following the gingival margin is indicative of plaque accumulation and a cariogenic diet (Figure 16.1Bii). Poor hygiene during orthodontic treatment predisposes to decalcification, gingival hyperplasia, periodontal breakdown and removable-appliance-related stomatitis.

Assessment of dental development

It is important to note the teeth present and the mobility of the deciduous teeth that are present. A mobile deciduous tooth often indicates eruption of the successor is occurring. The stage of dental development can be classified as follows:
- Deciduous dentition;
- Early mixed dentition – marked by eruption of the permanent incisors and first molars;
- Late mixed dentition – marked by eruption of all successional teeth excluding the second premolars;
- Permanent dentition.

The **chronological age** gives an indication of the teeth likely to be present within the mouth permitting for individual variation. Abnormalities in the **sequence of eruption** are more informative in detecting developmental disturbances (see Chapter 7). **Asymmetries in dental development**, particularly when ≥6 months, are also indicative of developmental disturbances and warrant radiographic assessment.

Developmental disturbances in **tooth size** are common (Figure 16.1C). The maxillary lateral incisor is often diminutive or peg shaped. Microdontia can be associated with hypodontia. Macrodontia is less common and can occur as an isolated phenomenon or in association with supernumerary teeth. **Tooth size (Bolton) discrepancies** can impact on aesthetics, especially when the maxillary lateral incisor is affected, and can influence how well the arches occlude following comprehensive orthodontic treatment.

Assessment of tooth position

The segments of each arch should be assessed in turn: (1) labial segments, (2) canines and (3) buccal segments.

It is important to quantify the amount of **crowding or spacing** within each segments and the **inclination** of the incisors and molars.

The inclination of the teeth is determined by a combination of skeletal and soft tissue factors. In Class II malocclusion, the lower incisors may be proclined (**dento-alveolar compensation**) if the soft tissues are favourable, to compensate for the anteroposterior skeletal discrepancy. Similarly in Class III malocclusion, the upper incisors may be proclined and the lowers retroclined (Figure 8.1A). The existence of an abnormal **frenal attachment** should always be considered in the presence of a diastema (Figure 9.1D).

Canine angulation is classified as mesial, upright or distal. Mesially angulated canines may upright spontaneously if the first premolars are extracted. Distally angulated canines can cause incisor proclination during alignment as their crown tends to be thrown forwards. It may then be anchorage demanding to retract the labial segment into its pre-treatment position particularly if space is also required to correct crowding.

In the presence of a transverse maxillary deficiency, the upper molars may be buccally inclined and the lowers lingually inclined to compensate for the transverse skeletal discrepancy. It is important to note the inclination of the upper molars because if they are already buccally inclined, further dental tipping may not be advisable for crossbite correction.

Static and dynamic occlusion

The following features should be noted in the intercuspal position:
- overjet, overbite and centreline relationships;
- incisor, canine and molar relationships;
- crossbites.

The **Angle classification** and the British Standards Institute **incisor classification** are summarised in Tables 10.1 and 10.2, respectively. The **overjet** is the horizontal distance between the labial surfaces of the mandibular incisors and the maxillary incisal edges. It should be measured parallel to the occlusal plane (normal = 2–4 mm) and to the most prominent point on the maxillary central incisal edges. If there is an anterior **mandibular displacement**, it is important to measure the overjet at initial contact before the displacement to obtain a true measure of the occlusal discrepancy. The **overbite** is the degree of vertical overlap of the mandibular incisors by their maxillary counterparts measured perpendicular to the occlusal plane (normal = 2–4 mm). The depth of the **curve of Spee** in the mandibular arch is related to the depth of the overbite. The overbite can be classified as complete or incomplete (see Chapter 27). If complete to gingival tissues, the presence and extent of gingival trauma should be noted. In cases of **anterior open bite**, an assessment should be made of the symmetry of the open bite, its vertical extent in millimetres and how far it extends distally.

The coincidence and angulation of the maxillary and mandibular **dental centrelines** should be compared with the midfacial line. The maxillary centreline should be coincident and parallel to the midfacial line for ideal aesthetics. The lower dental centreline has less importance aesthetically, but should be corrected to establish the correct buccal segment relationship.

If a **crossbite** is present, it is important to check for a mandibular displacement on closure (see Chapter 30). The site of premature contact and direction and magnitude of displacement should be noted. There may be excessive toothwear on the tooth making premature contact.

As well as the static occlusion, it is important to check for **occlusal interferences** during excursions of the mandible. These may predispose to temporomandibular joint dysfunction.

Path of mandibular closure

A **mandibular displacement** is a lateral or sagittal movement of the mandible from the rest position to the position of maximum intercuspation due to a premature occlusal contact. A displacement can result in a crossbite, change in overjet and centreline discrepancy depending on its direction. Orthodontic treatment should be planned to the retruded contact position.

A **mandibular deviation** is a sagittal movement of the mandible during closure from a **habitual posture** to maximum intercuspation. It is often seen in Class II division 1 malocclusion where the patient postures forwards to obtain a lip to lip oral seal and/or improve aesthetics. It is important that all records are taken in the intercuspal position for treatment planning.

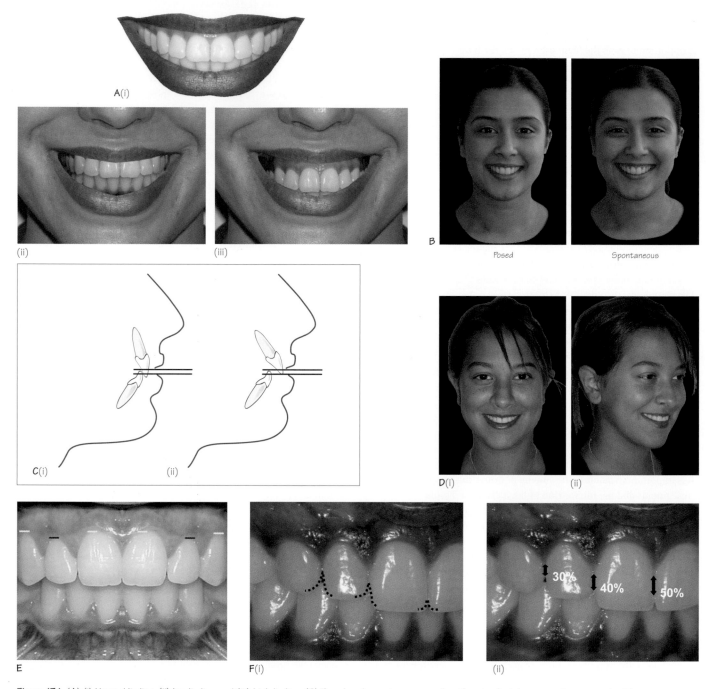

Figure 17.1 (**A**) (i) Normal lip line, (ii) low lip line and (iii) high lip line. (**B**) Posed and spontaneous smiles. Greater facial movements are required for the generation of the spontaneous smile which produces greater upper lip elevation and tooth/gingival exposure. (**C**) Proclination of the maxillary incisors results in a reduction of tooth display at rest and during smiling. Retroclination will have the opposite effect. (**D**) The smile arc is shown in red. (**E**) The ideal relationship of the anterior maxillary gingival margins. (**F**) the ideal (i) embrasure and (ii) connector relationship.

Most patients seek orthodontic treatment to improve their smile aesthetics. With modern orthodontic and restorative techniques, it is possible to improve the appearance of the smile, assuming its individual components are understood. Knowledge of these components is also important for informed consent, as any anatomical limitations in achieving ideal aesthetics should be explained before commencing treatment. This chapter discusses the **important components** of a smile.

The lip line

The lip line is the vertical relationship between the upper lip and the maxillary incisors during smiling. Ideally, the full length of the upper incisors and the interdental papillae should be visible during smiling. The lip line is high when a continuous band of gingival tissue is visible and low when less than 75% of the crown height of the central incisors can be seen (Figure 17.1A). The lip line in females is 1–2 mm higher than in males so it is acceptable for females to show 1–2 mm of gingivae anteriorly during smiling.

Many factors influence the lip line and amount of incisor display during rest and smiling:

(1) **The type of smile**. The **posed smile** is a **voluntary** smile, not linked with emotion, that is fairly reproducible. An example of a posed smile is the smile elicited when someone is asked to smile for a photograph. The **spontaneous smile** is an **involuntary** smile, linked with emotion, where there is maximal elevation of the upper lip (Figure 17.1B). An example of a spontaneous smile is the smile elicited when somebody is told a funny joke. It is important to assess both the posed and spontaneous smile during examination as the amount of incisor and gingival shown in the latter is greater.

(2) **Elevation of the upper lip**. There is individual variation in upper lip elevation during smiling (mean = 7–8 mm). Excessive elevation, also termed hypermobility, results in a high lip line.

(3) **Vertical maxillary height**. Vertical maxillary excess can result in a high lip line. Conversely, vertical maxillary deficiency, sometimes associated with maxillary retrognathia, can result in a low lip line. Orthognathic surgery can be used to treat such discrepancies.

(4) **Vertical dental height**. Reduced vertical dental height, as seen with digit sucking, results in reduced incisor display.

(5) **Incisor inclination**. Proclination of the maxillary incisors results in elevation of their incisal edges and a reduction in tooth display. Conversely, retroclination increases tooth display (Figure 17.1C).

The smile arc

The smile arc is the relationship between the curvature of the maxillary incisal edges and the curvature of the lower lip in the posed smile (Figure 17.1D). For ideal aesthetics, the maxillary incisal edges should lie parallel to the curvature of the lower lip. In such cases, the smile arc is termed **consonant**.

If the maxillary incisal edges do not run parallel to the lower lip or have a reverse curvature (e.g. in anterior open bite), the smile arc is termed **non-consonant**. The smile arc flattens with age because of toothwear. Poor orthodontic treatment, with incorrect positioning of the incisal edges, can also lead to flattening of the smile arc. Ideally, the incisal edges of the maxillary central incisors and the cusp tips of the canines should be at the same level in the horizontal plane whereas the incisal edges of the lateral incisors should be 1 mm apical to this level.

Tooth size and symmetry

A symmetrical dental arrangement is important in anterior dental aesthetics. In patients with missing anterior teeth, it is important to undertake **joint orthodontic-restorative planning** to plan space redistribution to ensure correct tooth size of missing units and symmetry.

Central incisors can appear short and broad if they have suffered trauma, undergone toothwear or when the gingival margin has failed to migrate apically with development. For ideal aesthetics, the width of the central incisor should be 80% of its length. Restorative dentistry and periodontal surgery can be used to optimise this ratio.

The midlines

The **facial midline** is a line extending from soft tissue nasion to the midpoint of the upper lip. Ideally, the **maxillary dental centreline** should be coincident and parallel to this. However, research suggests that parallelism is more important than coincidence. Aesthetically, the **mandibular midline** is not as important as the maxillary midline. However, it is important occlusally as good buccal interdigitation can only be achieved if the upper and lower midlines are coincident.

Buccal corridors

The width of the buccal corridor is the space between the buccal surface of the most distal maxillary molar and the angle of the mouth during smiling. Ideally, this should be minimal in order to give the smile a broad appearance. The buccal corridor depends on a number of factors:

• Arch width and archform. Increasing arch width will reduce the buccal corridor. For stability, the dental arches can only be expanded within acceptable limits.

• Anteroposterior maxillary position. As a wider part of the maxilla is moved forward with orthognathic surgery, the buccal corridor width reduces.

• Molar inclination. Palatally inclined premolar/molars increase the buccal corridor width.

• Inter-commissure distance during smiling. The greater this distance, the greater the buccal corridor width.

Gingival aesthetics

Ideally, the gingival margins of the maxillary central incisors and canines should be level whereas those of the lateral incisors should lie 1 mm more incisally (Figure 17.1E). The significance of gingival aesthetics is greatest when the lip line is high. Box 17.1 outlines factors that can result in gingival marginal discrepancies. Orthodontic intrusion and extrusion can be used to correct small discrepancies.

Box 17.1 Some causes of gingival margin discrepancies

• Periodontal disease
• Attrition
• Ankylosis in a growing patient
• Canines substituting as lateral incisors
• Severe crowding
• Delayed maturation of the gingival margin

Embrasures, connectors and contacts

Embrasures are the spaces between the incisal edges of adjacent teeth (Figure 17.1Fi). Ideally, embrasures should gradually increase in size from the maxillary central incisors, moving distally in the arch. Toothwear can result in elimination of embrasures, which results in an aged smile.

Connectors are the areas between adjacent teeth where they appear to meet. **Contacts** are the areas where they actually meet and are smaller than connectors. The connector between the central incisors should measure 50% of the height of the central incisor crown, between the central incisor and lateral incisor it should measure 40% of the length of the central incisor and between the lateral incisor and canine it should measure 30% of the length of the central incisor (**50–40–30 rule**; Figure 17.Fii). A poor connector relationship can result from incorrect angulation of adjacent teeth and/or a triangular tooth shape. The latter can be corrected by interproximal enamel reduction followed by orthodontic space closure.

18 Space analysis

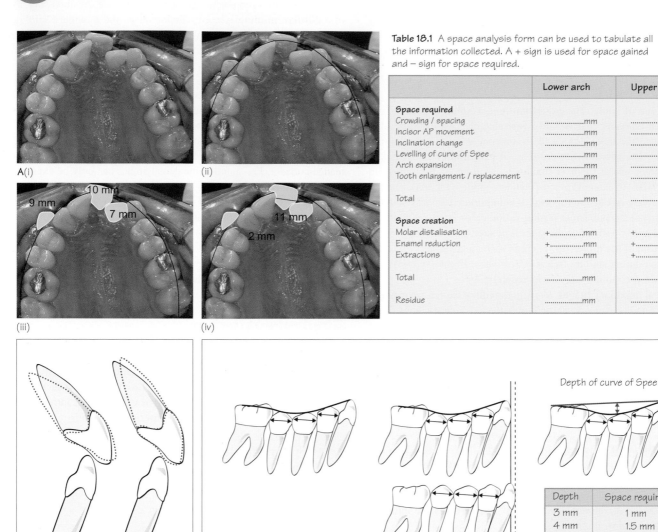

Table 18.1 A space analysis form can be used to tabulate all the information collected. A + sign is used for space gained and – sign for space required.

	Lower arch	Upper arch
Space required		
Crowding / spacing	....................mm	....................mm
Incisor AP movement	....................mm	....................mm
Inclination change	....................mm	....................mm
Levelling of curve of Spee	....................mm	....................mm
Arch expansion	....................mm	....................mm
Tooth enlargement / replacement	....................mm	....................mm
Total	....................mm	....................mm
Space creation		
Molar distalisation	+................mm	+................mm
Enamel reduction	+................mm	+................mm
Extractions	+................mm	+................mm
Total	................mm	................mm
Residue	................mm	................mm

Depth	Space required
3 mm	1 mm
4 mm	1.5 mm
5 mm	2 mm

Figure 18.1 (**A**) The assessment of dental crowding. (i) Pre treatment view of upper arch, (ii) an archform is constructed that fits the majority of teeth, (iii) the mesiodistal width of the crowded teeth is measured (9 + 10 + 7 = 26 mm), and (iv) the space available for alignment is measured (2 + 11 = 13 mm). The total arch crowding can then be calculated (26 – 13 = 13 mm). (**B**) Changes in incisor inclination affect space requirements. (i) Incisor proclination leads to an increase in overjet, and (ii) incisor retroclination can lead to a slight reduction in overjet. (**C**) (i) The curve of Spee consists of a series of slipped contact points in the vertical plane. (ii) Levelling of the curve of Spee involves aligning the contact points and requires space. (iii) the space required to level the curve of Spee is dependent on the depth of the curve.

The aim of space analysis is to determine the **space and anchorage requirements** for orthodontic treatment. The Royal London space analysis provides a comprehensive approach to space assessment.

Features of a malocclusion to consider in space analysis

(1) Crowding and spacing
Crowding and spacing should be measured mesial to the first permanent molars in relationship to the archform that fits the majority of teeth (Figure 18.1A). The mesiodistal width of the malaligned teeth is measured followed by the available space within the archform. **Crowding** can be quantified as **mild** (<4 mm), **moderate** (4–8 mm) or **severe** (≥8 mm).

If the second deciduous molars are retained, approximately 1 mm of space per quadrant will be available following exfoliation and eruption of second premolars in the upper arch and 2 mm in each quadrant in the lower arch. It is conventional to use a '**+**' sign for **space gained** and '**–**' sign for **space required**.

(2) Incisor anteroposterior movement

With few exceptions (see Chapter 11), the lower incisor anteroposterior (AP) position should be accepted to maximise stability. In Class II malocclusions, the upper incisors must be retracted for overjet reduction. Conversely, in Class III malocclusions the upper incisors may be advanced and the lowers retracted to correct a reverse overjet. For every 1 mm all four incisors are retracted, 2 mm of space (1 mm per quadrant) is required. Conversely, for every 1 mm all four incisors are advanced, 2 mm of space will be created.

(3) Changing inclination

Changing the inclination of the upper incisors has space implications. When they are actively proclined, the overjet increases and space is required to normalise this increase (Figure 18.1Bi). Approximately 1 mm of space is required to procline all four upper incisors by 5°. Conversely, when proclined incisors are retroclined, every 5° of retroclination will reduce the overjet by 0.5 mm, which reduces the space required for upper incisor retraction (Figure 18.1Bii).

(4) Levelling the curve of Spee

The curve of Spee is the curved line in the sagittal plane drawn along the cusps and incisal edges of the mandibular teeth (Figure 18.Ci). The curve consists of a series of slipped contact points in the vertical plane. A deep overbite can be reduced by levelling the curve of Spee. Levelling requires alignment of the contacts and has space implications (Figure 18.Cii).

The depth of the curve of Spee is measured at the greatest point from a line drawn between the distal cusps of the first molars and the incisal edges (Figure 18.1Ciii). Space is required to level the curve only if the overbite is deep and if the premolars have not been assessed as being crowded. The amount of space required per arch for different depths of the curve is shown in Figure 18.1Ciii.

(5) Arch expansion

Upper arch expansion is undertaken for crossbite correction and is useful in providing space for the relief of crowding and/or overjet reduction. Every 1 mm of expansion creates approximately 0.5 mm of space within the arch.

(6) Tooth enlargement or replacement

Mesiodistal enlargement of microdont teeth and replacement of missing teeth require space. This needs to be taken into account when determining total arch space requirements. A restorative opinion can advise on how much space is required as this depends on the final restoration planned.

Total space requirement

Once all of the above factors have been considered, it is possible to calculate the space required within each arch. Calculation is simplified if the information is tabulated as outlined in Table 18.1.

Space creation

The next factor to consider is how space will be created to fulfil the above objectives. Space can be created in several ways:

- use of leeway space;
- distal movement of the maxillary molars;
- arch expansion;
- incisor advancement;
- interproximal enamel reduction;
- extraction.

Use of **leeway space**, **arch expansion** and **incisor advancement** will have been considered when the total space requirement was calculated.

The amount of space gained from **distal maxillary molar movement** is dependent on the compliance of the patient and the amount of crowding distal to the upper first molars. If all factors are favourable, it is possible to distalise the upper molars by 6–7 mm per quadrant with headgear (see Figure 22.1D).

Interproximal enamel reduction is reserved for adults in whom the dental pulp has sufficiently migrated due to secondary dentine formation. It is most commonly undertaken in the lower labial segment where up to 3 mm of space can be created. Some clinicians may use this technique more extensively within the arch to create greater space. Bulky interproximal restorations can also be reduced in size to create space within the dental arch.

Dental **extractions** are a common technique for space creation once simpler methods have been excluded. Loss of a tooth with poor prognosis should be considered before a sound tooth is extracted, even if this may complicate treatment. Ideally, the teeth extracted should be close to the point of crowding. The first and second premolars are commonly extracted to provide space anteriorly. First premolar extractions provide more space anteriorly (40–65% of their width without anchorage reinforcement) than second premolar extractions (25–50%).

Determining anchorage requirements

Once the total space required and the space available has been calculated (Table 18.1), it is possible to determine the feasibility and anchorage requirements. If the space required is more than that created, the treatment is not feasible unless additional space is created or the treatment objectives are limited. If the space created is equal to or slightly more than the space required then **maximum anchorage** support (i.e. headgear, implants) is necessary. If more space will be created than is required, the residue will be taken up by mesial molar movement.

Effects of growth

Differential mandibular growth (see Chapter 4) can have space implications during treatment. It may be favourable in Class II malocclusion, depending on the direction of growth (see Chapter 5), as it aids overjet correction, molar correction (by mesial lower molar movement) and reduces space requirements for maxillary incisor retraction and molar correction. Conversely in Class III malocclusion, growth may reduce the overjet and move the molars in a Class III direction. This increases space requirements in the lower arch for incisor retraction. Although growth is impossible to predict, the prospect of an unfavourable growth pattern may influence an extraction decision particularly in Class III malocclusions.

Table 19.1 Radiation dose of some commonly used orthodontic investigations.

Radiograph	Total effective dose (mSv)	Equivalent of natural radiation (days)	Lifetime additional risk of cancer
Lateral ceph	0.1	14	1 in 200 000
DPT	0.016–0.026	2	1 in 1 000 000
Occlusal/periapical	0.008	1	1 in 10 000 000

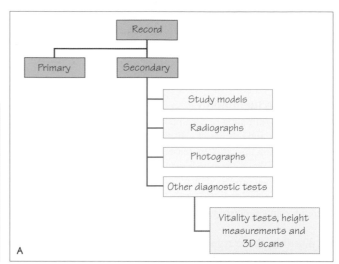

A

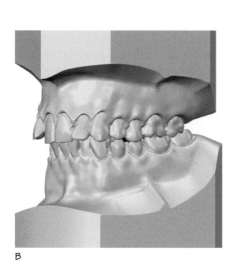

B

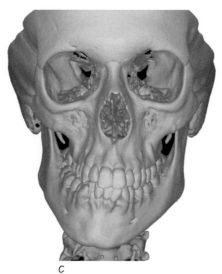

C

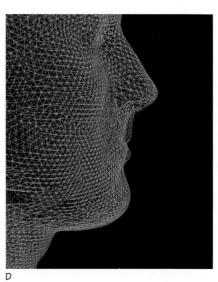

D

Figure 19.1 (A) A classification of orthodontic records. (B) Digital study model. The model can be rotated and viewed from all directions and measurements can be taken directly. (C) Cone beam computed tomography. The image can be viewed at different planes to assess the hard and soft tissues. (D) A 3D facial soft tissue scan showing the soft tissue profile before (white lines) and after (green lines) maxillary advancement surgery.

Records have a number of important functions in clinical practice. Box 19.1 lists the role of clinical records and Figure 19.1A provides a classification of records. The **primary record** is the written record and should include information such as patient demographics, relevant history, the findings of examination and special investigations, the diagnosis, treatment plan and a record of informed consent. It is also important to keep a record of treatment with the date and signature of the operator clearly marked. **Secondary records** are collected to aid diagnosis, monitor treatment and complement the primary record.

> **Box 19.1 Role of orthodontic records**
>
> - Diagnosis and treatment planning
> - Acting as an aide-memoire
> - Providing a legal document of treatment
> - Providing proof to commissioning bodies that treatment was justified and conducted to a good standard
> - Audit, teaching and research

Study models

Orthodontic study models are acquired at the beginning, sometimes during, and at the end of treatment. They should be fully extended into the buccal sulcus and record all the teeth present. **Angle's trimming** is undertaken to enable the occlusion to be examined at varying angles with the models placed on a flat surface. Study models have a number of uses including:

- treatment planning (e.g. space analysis);
- monitoring growth;
- monitoring treatment progress;
- patient education;
- diagnostic (Kesling's) set-ups;
- acting as a legal record;
- audit, research and teaching.

Digital study models (Figure 19.1B) eliminate the problems of storage and allow computerised analysis and may become widely used in the future.

There is no need to mount study models onto an **adjustable articulator** for routine orthodontic care. They are only mounted, using a facebow transfer, for orthognathic cases involving maxillary surgery.

Radiographs

A radiographic examination is only justified if the patient's management could be modified by the results. Table 19.1 outlines the radiation doses for some common radiographic investigations. Radiographs most commonly used in orthodontic practice include the:

- dental panoramic tomogram (DPT);
- lateral cephalogram;
- upper anterior occlusal view.

Additional films that are occasionally requested include periapical radiographs, bitewing radiographs and posteroanterior cephalometric views.

A **DPT** is often taken before treatment and near the end of fixed appliance treatment. In addition to identifying general and dental pathology, the DPT is useful for assessing dental development, localising unerupted teeth and assessing root length during diagnosis and treatment planning. It can be helpful near the end of treatment to assess root length and root parallelism. One major limitation is that the anterior maxillary region may not be clearly visible. In such cases, the DPT can be supplemented with **an upper anterior occlusal view**.

The uses of the **lateral cephalometric view** include:

- diagnosis and treatment planning;
- monitoring growth (serial radiographs);
- monitoring treatment changes (serial radiographs);
- monitoring stability following orthognathic surgery;
- assisting in the localisation of unerupted teeth;
- estimation of skeletal age by assessing development of the cervical vertebra;
- audit, research and teaching.

Cephalometry should not be a substitute for a detailed clinical examination. Occasionally the results of cephalometric analysis contradict clinical findings. If in doubt, greater credibility should be given to the results of clinical examination.

It is useful to **monitor growth** before orthognathic surgery. It is particularly important in Class III malocclusions to ensure facial growth has plateaued before attempting correction.

A lateral cephalometric view is often taken at the end of functional appliance treatment, during fixed appliance treatment before final space closure, and following orthognathic decompensation to **monitor treatment changes**. It is particularly useful to know about any changes in lower incisor anteroposterior (AP) position following functional appliance treatment and just before completing space closure with fixed appliances. With few exceptions (see Chapter 11), an aim of treatment is often to maintain

the lower incisor AP position. Comparison of sequential radiographs highlights proclination or retroclination, allowing adjustments in treatment mechanics to re-establish the pre-treatment incisor position.

A lateral cephalogram is not often taken specifically to locate the position of **unerupted teeth**. However, if the film is already available, it can assist in localising the bucco-palatal position of ectopic maxillary canines.

Periapical radiographs are useful for detailed examination of suspicious areas noted on a DPT, when monitoring root resorption, bone levels and for assessing root parallelism before implant placement.

The **posteroanterior cephalometric radiograph** is taken to assess facial asymmetry. A number of analyses, which are outside of the scope of this book, have been developed for its evaluation.

Digital radiographs are becoming increasingly popular. They have a number of advantages over conventional films including immediate viewing, reduction in radiation exposure and processing costs, and electronic storage and transmission.

Photographs

Extra-oral and intra-oral photographs are routinely taken at the start, sometimes during, and at completion of treatment. They provide a **colour record** of the condition of the hard and soft tissues (e.g. enamel hypoplasia). Photographs can be used for:

- treatment planning;
- monitoring growth;
- monitoring treatment progress;
- patient education;
- as a legal record and audit, research and teaching.

Serial height measurement

Serial height measurements can be useful for assessing the general state of development when planning treatment timing. Height measurements, plotted onto a **growth chart** (Figure 2.1D), can indicate the timing of the **adolescent growth spurt** for functional appliance treatment and provide an indication when growth is likely to be complete for orthognathic surgery.

Hand-wrist radiographs

The hand-wrist radiograph has been used to determine **skeletal age** by assessment of the pattern of ossification of the bones within the hand. There is limited clinical benefit of this technique and it has been abandoned by a number of clinicians.

Three-dimensional hard and soft tissue scans

Cone beam computed tomography (CBCT) is a technique that can be used for the generation of detailed three-dimensional (3D) images of both the hard and soft tissues (Figure 19.1C). The principal benefits over conventional CT include a 20% reduction in radiation exposure, the scans are quicker to acquire and the equipment is considerably cheaper. CBCT may be increasingly used in the future for the assessment of impacted teeth, skeletal discrepancies and the mandibular condyles.

3D facial soft tissue scans are increasingly being used to examine facial morphology, monitor growth and treatment progress (Figure 19.1D). Advantages include no radiation exposure and the soft tissues can be examined in three dimensions unlike conventional cephalometry. Scanning equipment is expensive and tends to be available only in larger hospitals.

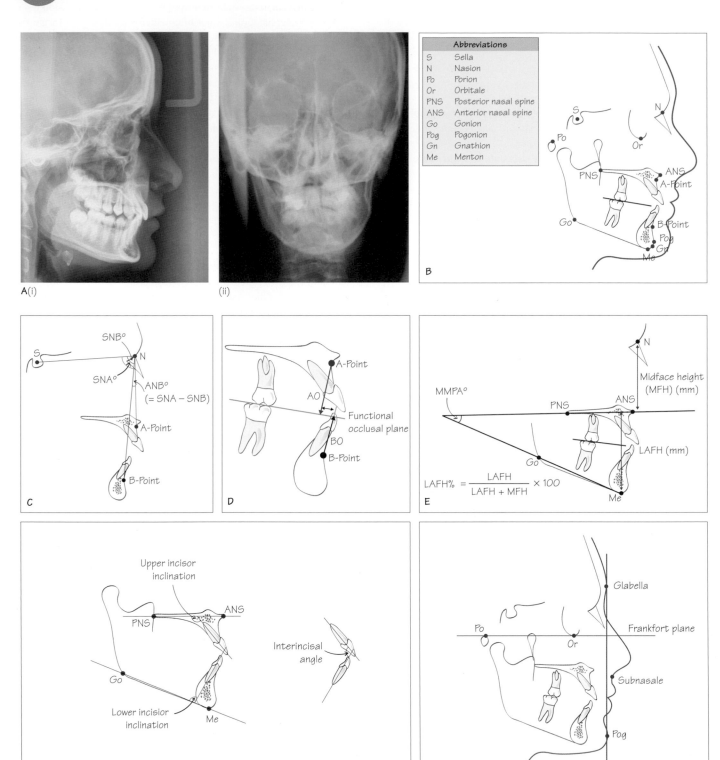

Figure 20.1 (**A**) (i) The lateral cephalogram. Note that the soft tissue outline is clearly visible and (ii) posteroanterior cephalogram of a patient with a mandibular asymmetry. (**B**) The main cephalometric points are summarised. For definitions please see Appendix 2. (**C**) Measurement of SNA, SNB and ANB. (**D**) The Wits analysis. (**E**) Assessment of the vertical dimension using MMPa and the lower anterior face height proportion (LAFH%). (**F**) Assessment of incisor inclinations and the interincisal angle. (**G**) Soft tissue analysis of maxillary and mandibular prominence.

Cephalometric radiography is a **standardised and reproducible** method of taking radiographs of the facial skeleton and cranial vault. The two cephalometric views used are the:

- **lateral cephalometric view** – the most commonly used and the focus of this chapter (Figure 20.1Ai);
- **posteroanterior cephalometric view** – used for the assessment of skeletal asymmetries (Figure 20.1Aii).

The **cephalostat** is a device used to standardise head position and magnification when taking cephalograms to enable comparison between sequential films. The vertical head position is standardised by placing ear posts into the external auditory meatus. The angulation of the head is standardised by ensuring that the Frankfort plane is parallel to the floor or the head is in the **natural head position** when the film is exposed. The magnification, usually between 5% and 12%, is kept constant by maintaining the x-ray tube to head distance (usually 150–180 cm (5–6 feet)) and head to film distance (usually 30 cm (1 foot)).

Lateral cephalometric analysis

Figure 20.1B shows the main cephalometric points and Appendix 2 lists the definitions of commonly used points and reference lines in alphabetical order. There are many hard tissue analyses and this chapter will focus on the principal components of cephalometric analysis.

Relationship of the maxilla and mandible to the cranial base

The anteroposterior (AP) position of the maxilla and mandible relative to the cranial base is represented by the angle **SNA** and **SNB**, respectively (Figure 20.1C). Table 20.1 outlines normal cephalometric values including SNA and SNB. An increased or decreased angle maybe due to protrusion or retrusion of the maxilla and mandible, respectively.

Table 20.1 Normal (Eastman) values for Caucasians unless stated otherwise*.

Measurement	Normal (SD)
SNA	81° (3°)
SNB	78° (3°)
ANB	3° (2°)
MMPA	27° (4°)
LAFH%	55% (2°)
U1–Maxillary plane	
Caucasians	109° (6°)
African Caribbeans•	118°
Chinese•	113°
L1–Maxillary plane	93° (6°)
Interincisal angle	135° (10°)

Relationship between the mandible and maxilla

Anteroposterior

The AP relationship between the mandible and the maxilla (i.e. the AP skeletal pattern) can be determined by measuring the angle **ANB** (= SNA − SNB). The skeletal pattern can be classified according to the following guidelines:

- ANB < 2°: Skeletal III pattern;
- 2° ≤ ANB ≤ 4°: Skeletal I pattern;
- ANB > 4°: Skeletal II pattern.

A major **limitation** of this approach is that changes in the position of nasion can alter angle ANB even if the relative position of the mandible and maxilla is maintained. If the angle between the maxillary plane and line S–N is within normal range (5–11°), the following adjustment, known as the **Eastman correction**, may help to compensate for this in Caucasians:

- 0.5° should be subtracted from ANB for every degree SNA is greater than 81°;
- 0.5° should be added to ANB for every degree SNA is less than 81°.

The **Wits analysis** also assesses the relative AP position of the mandible to the maxilla. It has the benefit of not involving the cranial base which eliminates problems created by incorrect positioning of nasion. The analysis compares the distance between perpendicular lines, drawn through point A (AO) and point B (BO), to the functional occlusal plane (Figure 20.1D). The normal distance between AO and BO should be:

- +1 mm (± 1.9 mm) in males;
- 0 mm (± 1.77 mm) in females.

Thus BO should be slightly ahead of AO (+ve) in males and coincident in females to indicate a skeletal I pattern. A skeletal II pattern is indicated when BO lies before AO (−ve) and vice versa for skeletal III. The main limitation of the Wits analysis is that the functional occlusal plane can be difficult to identify and its orientation may change with treatment which can affect measurements.

Vertical

The **maxillary-mandibular planes angle** (MMPA) and the **LAFH proportion** can be used to assess the vertical dimension (Figure 20.1E). An increased MMPA indicates an increased proportion between the LAFH and the posterior face height (i.e. ramus height). This is often due to an increased LAFH but may also be due to a reduced posterior face height. A reduced MMPA is most commonly due to a reduced LAFH but can also be caused by an increased posterior facial height. The ratio of the LAFH to the total face height gives an indication if the LAFH is within normal limits. Figure 20.1E illustrates how the LAFH% is calculated as a percentage of the total face height.

Incisor relationships

The angulation of the maxillary and mandibular incisors to the maxillary and mandibular plane, respectively, allows an assessment of incisor inclination (Figure 20.1F). The incisors maybe normally inclined, proclined or retroclined. The normal values for upper incisor inclination are given in Table 20.1. It is important to understand that there is **ethnic variation** in these normal values and that it is normal for African Caribbeans to have slightly greater proclination than Caucasians. The measured inclination of the lower incisors is not only influenced by the incisors but also by the inclination of the mandibular plane which is variable. The following formula, which takes into account the influence of the mandibular plane angle, can be used to calculate the normal lower incisor inclination for a given case:

Lower incisor inclination = 120°–MMPA

A normal interincisal angle is an important factor in preventing the relapse of deep overbite correction. Figure 20.1F outlines how this angle is measured.

Soft tissue analysis

Many soft tissue analyses exist and some useful measurements include:

- Measurement of the **nasolabial angle** (Figure 15.1B);
- Evaluating lip position relative to **Ricketts E-line** (Figure 15.1A);

• Evaluation of **maxillary and mandibular prominence** (Figure 20.1G). A line perpendicular to the Frankfort plane is drawn through glabella (see Appendix 2 for a definition). For assessment of maxillary position, subnasale should lie 6 ± 3 mm ahead of this line for facial balance. Regarding chin position, soft tissue pogonion should ideally lie 0 ± 4 mm behind the same line.

The management of malocclusion

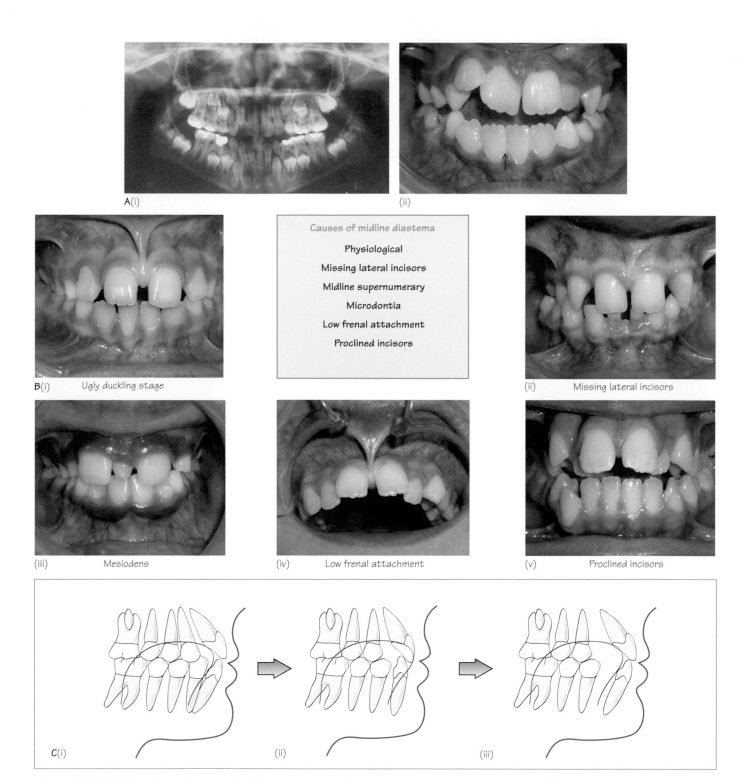

Figure 21.1 (**A**) (i & ii) Early loss of the lower right first deciduous molar has resulted in space loss for the eruption of the first premolar and a significant shift of the lower dental centreline. (**B**) (i–v) Causes of midline maxillary diastema. (**C**) Management of bimaxillary proclination by incisor retraction. (i) The incisors are in a position of soft tissue balance between the lips and tongue (Equilibrium theory). (ii) Extraction of premolars and incisor retraction moves these teeth outside the position of soft tissue balance such that following treatment (iii) they procline with reopening of extraction spaces.

Class I malocclusion is a term used to describe a malocclusion where the lower incisor edges occlude on or directly beneath the cingulum plateau of the upper incisors (British Standards Institute incisor classification, Chapter 10). The prevalence of Class I malocclusion is estimated to be approximately 50% among Caucasians.

Although there is no anteroposterior malrelationship, there may be discrepancies in the vertical and/or transverse dimension. The molar relationship is variable and is influenced by the underlying skeletal pattern and if there has been early loss of deciduous teeth. There may be crowding or spacing within the arches.

Aetiology of Class I malocclusion

Skeletal factors

The skeletal relationship may be Class I, II or III. This is because if there is a Class II or III pattern associated with a favourable soft tissue environment, **dento-alveolar compensation** can result in correction of the incisor relationship.

Vertically, the skeletal relationship is variable with a normal, increased or decreased lower anterior face height (LAFH) and Frankfort–Mandibular planes angle.

In the transverse dimension, there may be mandibular asymmetry and/or the maxillary arch may be constricted giving rise to a posterior crossbite.

Soft tissues

The soft tissues are not generally important in the aetiology of Class I malocclusion with the exception of patients with bimaxillary proclination. In such cases, the upper and lower incisors are proclined because the position of soft tissue balance has been moved forward by flaccid lip musculature and/or increased pressure from the tongue.

Local factors

Crowding is a common feature in Class I malocclusion and may be due to **dento-alveolar disproportion** or early loss of deciduous teeth. Early unilateral loss of deciduous teeth can result in centreline displacement (Figure 21.1A).

When there is crowding within the arches, teeth may become impacted. Excluding the third molars, the maxillary canines are the most frequently impacted teeth (see Chapter 32). It is also quite common to see premolars impacted due to early loss of deciduous teeth (see Chapter 31).

Spacing between the incisors before eruption of the maxillary canines is a normal developmental milestone (ugly duckling stage; see Chapter 7). This is usually self-correcting when the permanent maxillary canines erupt. A midline **diastema of ≥4 mm** is unlikely to resolve spontaneously. A diastema may also be due to a number of other reasons including microdontia (e.g. peg shaped lateral incisors), developmental absence of the maxillary lateral incisors, a midline supernumerary tooth and the presence of a low frenal attachment (Figure 21.1B). Such factors should be excluded in a patient presenting with a persistent diastema. A persistent diastema is more common in those of African Caribbean origin.

Treatment of Class I malocclusion

The management of Class I malocclusion usually involves the relief of **crowding** and alignment. In simple cases, alignment may occur by **spontaneous tooth movement** or with the aid of a **removable appliance**.

Spontaneous tooth movement is likely to occur if the displaced tooth is angled away from the extraction site. The tooth will then tend to upright under the influence of the soft tissues and contraction of scar tissue at the site of extraction. The majority of spontaneous tooth movement is likely to occur within the first 9 months after tooth loss. Spontaneous tooth movement is enhanced when growth is active and if there are no occlusal interferences to prevent movement. If there is severe crowding consideration should be given to **space maintenance** until the desired tooth movement has occurred. Often spaces are left if no active orthodontic treatment is undertaken which may be acceptable if they are poorly visible or if the patient is unconcerned.

In cases in which tooth angulations are not ideal for spontaneous movement, where there are rotations or if the patient wishes to achieve a high quality finish, consideration must be given to the use of **fixed appliances**. A formal **space analysis** (Chapter 18) should be undertaken to determine space and anchorage requirements before commencing treatment.

Patients presenting with **spacing** may be difficult to treat depending on the cause. Microdontia can be treated restoratively if there is adequate space available for tooth enlargement. Where the spacing is not ideal, consideration should be given to the use of fixed appliances to idealise spaces following joint orthodontic-restorative planning. A more difficult situation to deal with is spacing due to generalised microdontia. Options include restorative build up of teeth to close visible spaces or orthodontic redistribution of spaces to less visible areas of the dental arch. Orthodontic treatment to close all the spaces may result in significant retraction of the incisors unless anterior anchorage is reinforced (e.g. facemask). Long-term retention is essential for the maintenance of space closure. The management of hypodontia is outlined in Chapter 33.

A **low frenal attachment** may be the cause of a persistent diastema between the maxillary central incisors. In such cases there will be blanching of the palatal papilla on pulling the frenum which indicates a palatal attachment (Figure 9.1D). Further evidence of a low attachment is the presence of a small notch in the interdental bone between the incisors on an upper anterior occlusal radiograph. Opinions differ for the **timing of frenectomy** in relationship to orthodontic treatment. Some prefer to undertake the procedure before orthodontics as it is felt that access to the surgical site is greater. Others prefer to undertake surgery after diastema closure as stability may be improved by contraction of scar tissue. There is no evidence to favour any approach and it is probably sensible to undertake surgery before orthodontics if other surgery is planned particularly under general anaesthesia. **Long-term retention** will be required to maintain diastema closure.

Patients with **bimaxillary proclination** may present with concerns of dental or lip protrusion. As the incisors are likely to be in a position of soft tissue balance, care must be taken with planning extractions and orthodontic retraction as there is a significant risk of relapse and reopening of extraction spaces (Figure 21.1C). If there is crowding within the arches that may be contributing to incisor protrusion, extractions can be undertaken with care and one can consider limited retraction of the incisors. **Long-term retention** is sensible in such cases. If there is spacing within the arches, this can be redistributed to less visible areas of the mouth whilst accepting the incisor position.

22 Class II division 1 malocclusion

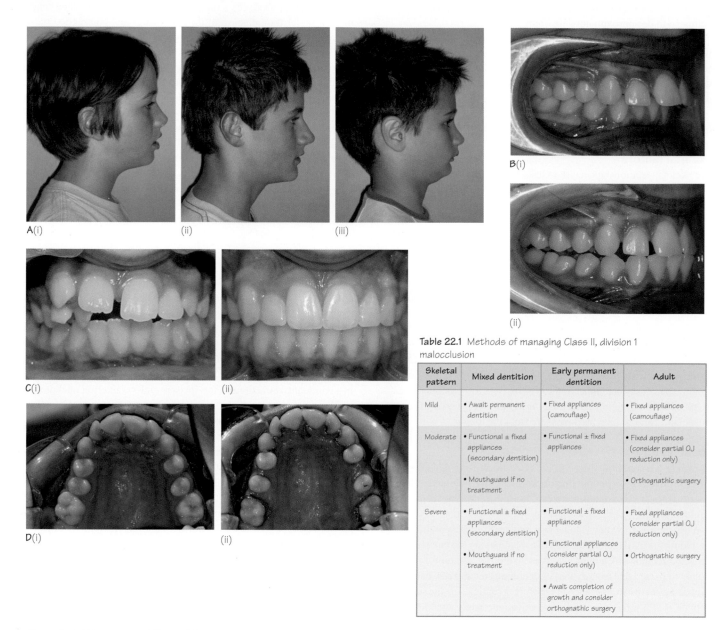

Figure 22.1 (**A**) Examples of (i) mild, (ii) moderate and (iii) severe Class II skeletal pattern due to mandibular retrognathia. (**B**) An example of a Class II, division 1 case treated with a functional (twin block) appliance for nine months: (i) start, (ii) end of twin block phase (note the reduction in overjet). (**C**) Class II, division 1 case treated by upper incisior retraction (orthodontic camouflage) using fixed appliances: (i) before and (ii) after treatment. (**D**) Case where space was created in the upper arch, for incisor retraction, with the use of headgear: (i) before and (ii) after headgear.

Table 22.1 Methods of managing Class II, division 1 malocclusion

Skeletal pattern	Mixed dentition	Early permanent dentition	Adult
Mild	• Await permanent dentition	• Fixed appliances (camouflage)	• Fixed appliances (camouflage)
Moderate	• Functional ± fixed appliances (secondary dentition) • Mouthguard if no treatment	• Functional ± fixed appliances	• Fixed appliances (consider partial OJ reduction only) • Orthognathic surgery
Severe	• Functional ± fixed appliances (secondary dentition) • Mouthguard if no treatment	• Functional ± fixed appliances • Functional appliances (consider partial OJ reduction only) • Await completion of growth and consider orthognathic surgery	• Fixed appliances (consider partial OJ reduction only) • Orthognathic surgery

Class II division 1 is the term used to describe a malocclusion in which the lower incisal edges lie posterior to the cingulum plateau of the upper incisors, the overjet (OJ) is increased and the upper incisors are normally inclined or proclined (British Standards Institute incisor classification, see Chapter 10). The molar relationship is often Class II, however, it may be Class I if there has been early loss of a lower deciduous molar and the first molar has drifted forwards. The overbite (OB) is variable but is often deep.

The **prevalence** of Class II division 1 malocclusion is 15–20% among Caucasians.

Aetiology of Class II division 1 malocclusion

Skeletal factors

Class II division 1 malocclusion is commonly accompanied by a **skeletal II pattern** with varying degrees of **mandibular retrognathia** (Figure 22.1A). Rarely, **maxillary protrusion** may be the primary aetiological factor. The vertical dimension is often normal or increased but can be decreased. If the soft tissues are favourable, the lower incisors are often proclined (**dento-alveolar compensation**) to compensate for the anteroposterior (AP) skeletal discrepancy (Figure 8.1A).

Habits and soft tissue factors

The presence of **incompetent lips**, with failure of the lower lip to control the position of the upper incisors, can be an important aetiological factor. The lips may be incompetent due to many reasons (Figure 15.1E). An **adaptive oral seal** is formed which may further influence incisor position. Lip to lip contact maybe possible by habitual forward posturing of the mandible and/or increased circumoral muscular activity. This helps in controlling the position of the upper incisors which may appear normally inclined. If there is a lip to palate anterior seal (termed a **lower lip trap**, Figure 8.1E), the soft tissues encourage upper incisor proclination and limit lower incisor proclination. Where the tongue contacts the lower lip to produce an anterior oral seal, the lower incisors are often proclined and the OB is *just* incomplete. Occasionally, a patient will have a very active lower lip, termed a **strap-like lower lip**, which causes retroclination of the lower incisors and exacerbates the Class II division 1 relationship. A **primary endogenous tongue thrust** (see Chapter 15) may also cause incisor proclination and lead to a Class II division 1 incisor relationship. Finally, **digit sucking** (see Chapter 9) can be an important factor in the aetiology of Class II division 1 malocclusion. It is important that habits are stopped before treatment is commenced.

Local factors

Crowding in the maxillary arch can exacerbate an increased OJ by causing further labial exclusion of the maxillary central incisors. Anterior **mandibular extractions**, especially during the mixed and early permanent dentition, can lead to uprighting of the lower incisors under lip pressure and an increase in OJ and OB.

Treatment of Class II division 1 malocclusion

Benefits of treatment include:

- an improvement in dento-facial aesthetics;
- a reduction in the risk of traumatic dental injuries. The risk of trauma increases as the OJ increases (see Chapter 12) particularly when the lips are incompetent;
- Relief of a deep traumatic OB (Chapter 27).

The treatment of Class II division 1 (Table 22.1) depends on the patient's motivation, age, severity of skeletal discrepancy and the facial profile.

Mixed dentition

Functional appliance treatment (see Chapter 39) is often undertaken in **moderate** Class II cases in the *late* mixed dentition so that fixed appliances can be placed immediately following AP correction (Figure 22.1B). However, treatment *can* be undertaken earlier if the **psychological impact** of the malocclusion is significant or if the **risk of trauma** is considered to be large. A prolonged retention period is then required until the permanent dentition has established and fixed appliances can be placed. Such long-term treatment may introduce problems with patient compliance. **Severe** Class II cases can be managed with functional appliances, however, large facial changes should not be expected. A **mouthguard** can be prescribed to reduce the risk of dental trauma during sports if treatment is not commenced at this stage. **Mild** Class II cases should be managed in the permanent dentition when a full fixed appliance can be placed.

Permanent dentition

In the permanent dentition, **mild** cases can be treated with **fixed appliances** by upper incisor retraction (camouflage treatment, Figure 22.1C). Before fixed appliances are placed, space often has to be created for the relief of crowding and/or upper incisor retraction. If the lower arch is well aligned, **headgear** can be used to retract the upper molars into a Class I position (Figure 22.1D). The choice of high, combined or low-pull headgear should be based on the vertical dimension (see Chapter 37). If the patient does not wish to wear headgear, or compliance is poor, **upper premolars** can be extracted to provide space assuming all other teeth are sound and present. Depending on the space requirements, **anchorage** may need to be reinforced with headgear (maximum anchorage) or a Nance palatal arch. If there is sufficient crowding in the lower arch, teeth can be extracted to provide space. A common **extraction pattern** is the loss of upper first and lower second premolars as the anchorage balance favours upper incisor retraction and mesial movement of the lower molar to facilitate Class II molar correction. Anchorage can be reinforced, if necessary, using **Class II intermaxillary traction**, which favours mesial movement of the lower molar and retraction of the upper incisors, or headgear. This extraction pattern should not be assumed for all cases as it depends on space requirements, the presence and condition of the remaining teeth and the facial profile.

Moderate Class II cases are often best managed with **functional appliances** to reduce the OJ, followed by fixed appliances for alignment. Alternatively, **fixed appliances** alone, often with **headgear** support, can be used to camouflage the skeletal discrepancy by upper incisor retraction. If the lower labial segment is retroclined, due to a lip trap, thumb sucking habit or trapping of the incisors by a deep OB, slight advancement can be considered without compromising stability significantly (see Chapter 11). If full retraction of the upper incisors is likely to be detrimental to **upper lip support**, for example when the nasolabial angle is obtuse (Figure 11.1C) and the lips are behind Ricketts E-line, consideration should be given to alignment only or **partial OJ correction** to maintain upper lip support. If at all possible, extractions should be avoided in such cases as there is a **risk of relapse** if the incisors are not fully retracted behind the lower lip with a consequent reopening of extraction spaces. In such cases, spacing already present between the incisors, or created following the use of headgear, should be used. The need for **long-term retention** should be emphasized during the consenting stage in such cases.

Severe Class II malocclusion may be managed with **functional appliances** during the early permanent dentition unless the patient is very concerned about their facial appearance. In such cases, the malocclusion is best managed at the completion of facial growth with a combination of orthodontics and **orthognathic surgery**. If, for whatever reason, surgery is not an option or the patient can not tolerate functional appliances, an improvement in aesthetics may be achieved with alignment only and/or **partial OJ reduction** using fixed appliances.

Stability of Class II correction

Relapse of Class II correction can be related to:

- positioning the upper incisors out of control of the lower lip and non-attainment of a lip to lip anterior oral seal (Figure 15.1Fi);
- relapse of excessively proclined lower incisors;
- unfavourable AP and vertical skeletal growth especially if associated with a clockwise (backward) mandibular growth rotation (see Chapter 5);
- continuation of a digit-sucking habit.

Class II division 2 malocclusion

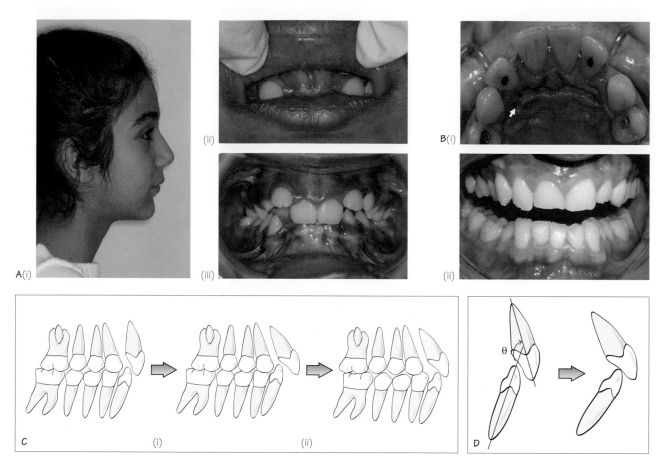

Figure 23.1 (**A**) *Some features of Class II, division 2 malocclusion: (i) mild mandibular retrognathia, with a pronounced chin point and reduced lower anterior face height, (ii) high lower lip line, and (iii) retroclined maxillary central incisors and deep overbite. (**B**) Traumatic overbite leading to (i) periodontal damage on the palatal aspect of the upper right lateral incisor and (ii) severe attrition. (**C**) The management of Class II, division 2 malocclusion with functional appliances involves (i) proclining the maxillary incisors into a Class II, division 1 relationship, which allows forward posturing of the mandible, and (ii) correction of the overjet. (**D**) Reduction of an increased interincisal angle is important for stable overbite correction.*

Class II division 2 is the term used to describe a malocclusion where the lower incisal edges occlude posterior to the cingulum plateau of the upper incisors and the upper central incisors are retroclined (British Standards Institute classification). The overbite (OB) is characteristically deep, the overjet maybe normal or increased, and the molar relationship is Class II. There is an association between this malocclusion and **impacted maxillary canines**. The **prevalence** of Class II division 2 is estimated to be approximately **10%** among Caucasians. This malocclusion has a strong genetic association.

Aetiology of Class II division 2 malocclusion

Skeletal factors

Class II division 2 is commonly associated with a **mild skeletal II pattern** due to mandibular retrognathia. The chin point may be

well positioned in a number of cases with retrusion more evident at the dento-alveolar region (Figure 23.1Ai). A moderate/severe skeletal II pattern may be present, however, is more likely to be associated with a Class II division 1 incisor relationship as the lips are more likely to be incompetent. Class II division 2 may rarely be associated with a skeletal I or III relationship if the soft tissue pattern is unfavourable.

Vertically, the lower anterior face height (LAFH) and Frankfort–Mandibular planes angle is often **reduced** (Figure 23.1Ai). This may be associated with an anticlockwise (forward) mandibular growth rotation (see Chapter 5). A reduction in the LAFH predisposes to a high lower lip line, deep OB and a pronounced labiomental fold.

In the **transverse** dimension, there may be a **scissor bite** in the premolar region which is a result of narrowing of the lower arch and because a wider part of the maxilla opposes a narrower part of the mandible (relative transverse discrepancy, Chapter 8).

Soft tissue factors

As a result of the reduced LAFH, the lower lip usually rests high on the crowns of the maxillary central incisors (Figure 23.1Aii). A **high lower lip line** results in retroclination of the maxillary central incisors, an increase in interincisal angle and deepening of the OB (Figure 23.1Aiii).

A deep **labiomental fold** is often seen in this malocclusion and reflects the relative soft tissue lip abundance due to a reduced LAFH.

Class II division 2 may result from retroclination of all the upper and the lower incisors (**bimaxillary retroclination**), caused by **strap-like lips** (Chapter 8), irrespective of the skeletal pattern.

Local factors

As well as a reduced LAFH, factors contributing to deep OB include an **increased interincisal angle**, sometimes due to retroclination of both upper *and* lower incisors, and occasionally a poorly developed maxillary incisor **cingulum** plateau which fails to prevent lower incisor over-eruption. An increased interincisal angle can lead to over-eruption of both upper and lower incisors. Over-eruption and retroclination of the upper incisors may contribute to the development of a **gummy smile**.

The **lower incisors** maybe **retroclined** because a deep OB can trap them within the palate and/or because of increased lip activity. Crowding is often associated with retroclined incisors. As well a trapping the lower incisors, a deep OB may confine the lower canines and premolars predisposing to a reduction in lower intercanine width and scissor bite in the premolar regions, respectively.

The maxillary **lateral incisors** are often **proclined** relative to the central incisors, mesially tipped and rotated. This may be a reflection of crowding (dento-alveolar disproportion) and/or because the lower lip fails to control the shorter lateral incisor crown.

Treatment of Class II division 2 malocclusion

Benefits of treatment include:
- improvement in dento-facial aesthetics;
- correction of a traumatic OB – a deep OB may be traumatic to the gingiva palatal to the maxillary incisors (Figure 23.1Bi), labial to the mandibular incisors and may predispose to incisor attrition (Figure 23.1Bii).

There are a number of **treatment approaches** for the correction of Class II division 2:
- functional appliances followed by fixed appliances;
- fixed appliances;
- orthodontics with orthognathic surgery.

Functional appliances (see Chapter 39) are useful in growing children with moderate or severe mandibular retrognathia, a reduced LAFH, deep OB and Class II molars. Before commencing treatment, it is often necessary to correct the inclination of the maxillary incisors to allow forward posturing of the mandible during the functional appliance phase. This essentially involves converting the Class II division 2 into a Class II division 1 malocclusion with the use of an upper removable appliance or an upper anterior fixed appliance (Figure 23.1C). The main advantage of using a functional appliance is that it reduces the anchorage requirements of later fixed appliance treatment by reducing the overjet, correcting the molar relationship and reducing the OB.

Following the functional appliance phase, which usually lasts 9–12 months, a period of fixed appliance treatment is often commenced for final alignment. This may be undertaken on an extraction or non-extraction basis depending on the space requirements of the case. It maybe prudent to supplement anchorage with headgear if treatment is undertaken on a non-extraction basis.

In milder cases, and in patients past the pubertal growth spurt, treatment maybe provided with **fixed appliances** alone. If the lower arch is well alignment, or where there is scope for lower incisor proclination for the relief of crowding (see Chapter 11), treatment maybe undertaken on a **non-extraction** basis with the use of **headgear** to retract the upper molars into a Class I relationship. In those unwilling to wear headgear, an alternative is to extract two premolars in the upper arch. Problems encountered during treatment include difficulties in OB reduction and full correction of the maxillary central incisor inclination. OB correction is facilitated by non-extraction treatment, as the likelihood of incisor retraction is reduced by using an anterior bite plane and by incorporating the second molars into the fixed appliance at an early stage.

The decision to **procline the lower incisors** and expand the lower inter-canine width depends on whether normal lower arch development has been affected by the OB. This can be assumed if the OB is deep, the lower incisors are upright and the canines are lingually displaced. **Long-term retention** is important in cases where the AP incisor position is altered (Chapter 11).

In cases where there is a large space requirement, an **extraction approach** maybe necessary in both arches. An extraction pattern that may be applicable to a number of cases, but not all, is the loss of upper first and lower second premolars. In such cases, the anchorage balance favours minimal retraction of the lower incisors, mesial movement of the lower molars (which aids molars correction), retraction of the maxillary incisors and reduced mesial movement of the upper molars. It is important that the lower incisors are not retroclined as this leads to a further increase in OB.

Orthodontics in association with **orthognathic surgery** (Chapter 43) is necessary in non-growing patients with severe anteroposterior and vertical skeletal discrepancies. The decision to undergo this treatment is dependent on a **risk–benefit analysis**. Surgical risks include those associated with general anaesthesia, damage to the inferior dental nerve, and infection. Risks associated with orthodontics are outlined in Chapter 12. **Presurgical orthodontics** involves decompensation of incisor inclinations, alignment and transverse arch co-ordination. The most common surgical procedure is mandibular advancement with a bilateral sagittal split osteotomy. A reduction genioplasty maybe required in those cases where mandibular advancement unacceptably increases the chin prominence. In those with a reduced LAFH, the vertical dimension can be increased by levelling the curve of Spee following surgery by molar extrusion. If the LAFH is normal or increased, the OB can be reduced by a lower labial segment set-down.

Stability of Class II division 2 correction

The stability of Class II division 2 correction depends on:
- correction of the interincisal angle to maintain stability of OB correction by providing an occlusal stop for the mandibular incisors (Figure 23.1D);
- avoiding excessive lower incisor proclination;
- favourable mandibular growth – a anti-clockwise (forward) mandibular growth rotation can result in relapse of deep OB correction.

Table 24.1 Factors determining the management of Class III malocclusion.

Factor	Notes
Patient concerns	Dental concerns can be managed with orthodontics alone. Facial and/or functional concerns will often require orthognathic surgery
Motivation for treatment	Good dental health and motivation are required for complex treatment
Severity of skeletal discrepancy	A mild/moderate skeletal discrepancy may be treated with orthodontic camouflage particularly if the patient can achieve incisor edge-to-edge occlusion. A severe discrepancy can only be treated comprehensively with orthodontics and orthognathic surgery
Remaining growth	A malocclusion at the borerline of orthodontic correction before the pubertal growth spurt is likely to deteriorate with differential mandibular growth
Degree of dento-alveolar compensation	Pre-existing dento-alveolar compensation limits the amount of further compensation achievable by orthodontic camouflage
Ability to achieve edge-to-edge bite	An ability to achieve edge-to-edge favours orthodontic camouflage as it indicates that less incisor movement is required for correction than suggested by the size of reverse overjet in centric occlusion
Depth of overbite	A deep overbite offers scope for camouflage by downwards and backwards rotation of the mandible (e.g. facemask) and improves stability of anterior crossbite correction

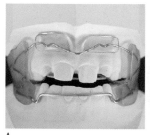
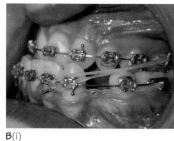
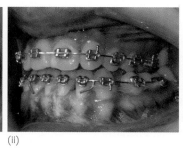
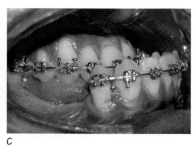

A   B(i)   (ii)   C

Figure 24.1 (**A**) The functional regulator III appliance. (**B**) An example of orthodontic camouflage. (i) Note use of Class III intermaxillary elastics to retract the lower incisors using the upper arch as anchorage (ii) after anterior crossbite correction. (**C**) Patient treated by alignment only as there were no facial concerns.

Class III is the term used to describe a malocclusion where two or more of the lower incisal edges occlude anterior to the cingulum plateau of the upper incisors (British Standards Institute incisor classification). The overjet (OJ) is reduced or reversed and there may be an anterior mandibular displacement. The molar relationship is often Class III.

The prevalence of Class III malocclusion shows **ethnic variation**. It is less common in Caucasians (prevalence 3%) than in the Japanese (5–10%).

Aetiology of Class III malocclusion

Skeletal factors

Class III malocclusion is commonly accompanied by a **skeletal III pattern** due to many possible factors including:

- increased mandibular length;
- forward positioning of the glenoid fossa;
- reduced maxillary length;
- short cranial base;
- reduced cranial base angle (Figures 3.1D and 3.1E);
- a combination of the above factors.

Rarely, this malocclusion can occur in association with a skeletal I or II pattern if the soft tissue environment is unfavourable. With favourable soft tissues, a skeletal III discrepancy may be compensated by upper incisor proclination and lower incisor retroclination (**dento-alveolar compensation**). In such cases, the OJ will not truly reflect the skeletal discrepancy. The **vertical dimension** is often increased, however, it can be reduced or normal. Unilateral or bilateral posterior **crossbites** can be found and may be due to a number of reasons: a narrow maxilla, a broad mandible or anterior-posterior (AP) skeletal discrepancy (relative transverse deficiency; Figure 8.1C). The upper molars maybe inclined buccally and the lower molars lingually to help compensate for the transverse discrepancy.

A severe skeletal III pattern can be associated with a cleft palate and a number of **craniofacial syndromes** (e.g. Crouzon's syndrome). Such patients should be treated in a multidisciplinary setting by dedicated craniofacial teams.

Growth is often unfavourable in Class III malocclusion because of **differential mandibular growth** (see Chapter 5). This leads to deterioration of the occlusal relationship once **dento-alveolar adaptation** (see Glossary) has reached its limits. This effect is greater in males than females and in those with a family history of mandibular prognathism.

Soft tissue factors

The soft tissues do not have as big a role in the aetiology of Class III malocclusion as in other malocclusions. If the soft tissues are favourable, they encourage **dento-alveolar compensation** both in the AP and transverse dimensions. Occasionally, the **tongue** is large and adopts a lower than normal resting position. This can lead to a broader lower arch, exacerbating any posterior crossbite tendency and proclination of the lower incisors, which worsens the Class III incisor relationship.

Local factors
As the maxilla can be small and the mandible large, the upper arch is often crowded and the lower arch is well aligned or spaced.

Treatment of Class III malocclusion
Benefits of treatment include:
- An improvement in dento-facial aesthetics.
- Elimination of a mandibular displacement that may be associated with attrition at the site of premature contact, later temporomandibular joint dysfunction and strain of the lower incisor periodontal attachment in the case of an anterior crossbite.
- An improvement in function – severe Class III malocclusion may be associated with difficulty in mastication, particularly if there is an anterior open bite. With severe maxillary retrusion it may occasionally be beneficial to advance the maxilla to increase the size of the airway if there is evidence of obstructive sleep apnoea.

Class III malocclusion is the **least predictable** malocclusion to manage because of the uncertainty surrounding future growth. Successful treatment depends on a number of factors (Table 24.1).

In the **early mixed dentition**, upper incisor proclination can be considered for an anterior crossbite associated with a forward mandibular displacement. This can be achieved with an **upper removable appliance** or a simple fixed appliance (Chapter 38). A positive overbite is essential for post-treatment stability of crossbite correction. An anterior crossbite during the **late mixed dentition** can be treated by several approaches. If there is maxillary retrusion with a deep overbite and the patient is motivated, treatment can be undertaken using a **facemask** (see Figure 37.1Biv). The technique requires strict patient compliance as the facemask must be worn 10–12 hours/day for at least 6 months. The effects of facemask treatment include: forward maxillary movement, proclination of the maxillary incisors, downwards and backwards mandibular rotation and retroclination of the mandibular incisors. The skeletal effects are larger in patients younger than 10 years of age, and may be enhanced when **rapid maxillary expansion** is used concurrently. It is controversial whether this form of treatment leads to any long-term growth enhancement. Alternative treatment approaches less frequently used include use of a **chin cup** for mandibular protrusion and functional regulator III (Figure 24.1A) or a reverse twin block **functional appliance**. Correction with these techniques is mainly achieved by downwards and backwards mandibular rotation as well as lower incisor retroclination. Therefore these treatments are ideally indicated in patients with a deep overbite associated with a reduced vertical dimension.

During the **early permanent dentition**, if the skeletal discrepancy is **mild/moderate** one may consider **orthodontic camouflage** by upper incisor proclination and/or lower incisor retroclination, with the use of fixed appliances with or without extractions. The decision to commence treatment at this stage can be difficult particularly because of the uncertainly surrounding future growth. If the patient can achieve edge-to-edge incisor contact in centric relation, and there is no significant dento-alveolar compensation already present, commencing treatment at this stage may be considered. The decision to **extract** mainly depends on the degree of crowding present, the amount of lower incisor retraction required, the amount of upper incisor proclination allowable and an estimation of future growth. The amount of lower incisor retraction required will be influenced by the amount and direction of future mandibular growth. If there is a **severe** skeletal discrepancy during the early permanent dentition stage, one should await further growth and finally treat using a joint **orthognathic** approach. Growth can be monitored using serial study models, cephalograms and standing height measurements. If there is severe upper arch crowding and the patient is concerned, a short course of early fixed appliance treatment can be suggested to align the arches whilst awaiting further growth.

As already mentioned, the difficulty with undertaking treatment early is the uncertainty surrounding future mandibular growth. A **potential complication** that early treatment can create, particularly if it involves extractions, is that if growth is unfavourable and the patient decides to have orthognathic surgery at a later date, any camouflage treatment will have to be reversed in preparation for surgery (see Chapter 43). This may involve reopening previous extraction spaces with resultant restorative implications. If there is any major concern during the early permanent dentition stage regarding future mandibular growth, it is better to delay treatment until after the pubertal growth spurt when the effects of growth are better understood. A family history of severe Class III malocclusion increases the probability of unfavourable future growth.

In the **permanent dentition**, mild/moderate Class III malocclusion can often be treated with **orthodontic camouflage** (Figure 24.1B). Severe Class III malocclusion, and patients with moderate Class III malocclusion and facial concerns are best treated with orthodontics in combination with **orthognathic surgery**. The surgical treatment depends on which jaw(s) is contributing to the skeletal discrepancy. In very severe cases of maxillary retrusion (e.g. syndromes), **distraction osteogenesis** (see Chapter 44) may be necessary to achieve larger amounts of skeletal movement. Sometimes a patient with a severe discrepancy is happy to undergo **alignment only**, accepting the underlying skeletal discrepancy, if there are no facial concerns (Figure 24.1C).

Stability of Class III correction
Relapse of Class III correction may be related to:
- An **inadequate overbite** to maintain the corrected incisor position.
- **Unfavourable growth** in the AP and vertical skeletal dimension. Unfavourable AP growth can result in a relapse of overjet correction whereas unfavourable vertical growth can result in a reduction of overbite.

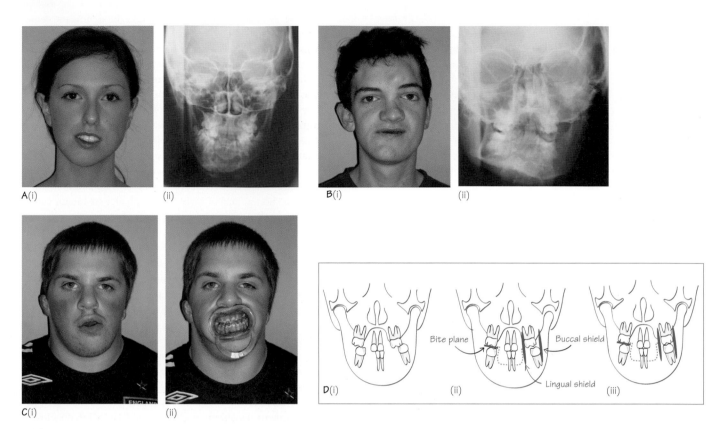

Figure 25.1 (**A**) A case of left-sided hemimandibular elongation. Note the significant lateral displacement of the chin point towards the unaffected side. (**B**) A case of left-sided hemimandibular hyperplasia. Note the extensive vertical component of growth, with minimal displacement of the chin point, and a twisted appearance to the chin. (**C**) (i) A patient with left sided hemifacial microsomia. (ii) Note the severe cant in the maxillary occlusal plane due to underdevelopment of the left side mandibular ramus. (**D**) The use of a hybrid functional appliance to maximise growth. (i) A left-sided mandibular deficiency with resultant displacement of the chin point, dental centreline and maxillary occlusal cant. (ii) Insertion of a hybrid functional appliance constructed with the centrelines corrected and left condyle distracted. A bite plane is used to prevent eruption of the right molars whilst disocclusion encourages eruption of the left molars. The lingual shield prevents interpostion of the tongue that may limit eruption and the buccal shield encourages unilateral expansion. (iii) The desired end result.

Symmetry is defined as correspondence in size, shape and relative position of parts on opposite sides of a median plane. The facial midline is usually taken as a line passing through soft tissue nasion and the midpoint of the upper lip. A degree of facial asymmetry is normal and acceptable across this line. It can be caused by an asymmetry in the facial **skeleton** and/or **soft tissue** drape. The point at which an asymmetry becomes unacceptable is when an individual begins to have aesthetic concerns and/or functional limitations. There is individual variation regarding when this point is reached. Although asymmetries can occur at many levels of the face, this chapter will mainly focus on developmental asymmetries affecting the mandible and maxilla. Table 25.1 provides a **classification** of asymmetries.

Developmental causes

Hemimandibular elongation and hyperplasia
Hemimandibular elongation is a developmental deformity, of unknown aetiology that usually affects one side of the mandible

Table 25.1 Classification of mandibular/maxillary asymmetries based on aetiology.

Cause	Examples
Developmental	Hemimandibular elongation and hyperplasia
	Hemifacial microsomia
	Hemimandibular atrophy
	Hemifacial hypertrophy
	Torticollis
	Hemifacial atrophy (Parry–Romberg syndrome)
Pathological	Infection
	Tumours
	Cysts
	Condylar resorption
Traumatic	Mandibular/maxillary fractures
	Post irradiation
Functional	Mandibular displacement (lateral component)

and presents with a progressively increasing **transverse** displacement of the chin that often becomes apparent during or after the adolescent growth spurt (Figure 25.1A). The mandibular dentition follows the skeletal displacement, which predisposes to buccal crossbite and centreline displacement away from the affected side and a scissor bite on the affected side. Since there is a *minimal* vertical component to the abnormal growth pattern, there is typically no over-eruption of the maxillary dentition on the affected side.

In contrast to hemimandibular elongation, **hemimandibular hyperplasia** presents with **transverse** *and* **vertical** enlargement of one side of the mandible during adolescence. As a consequence of the vertical component of abnormal growth, the height on the affected side of the face is increased. The dentition on that side over-erupts to maintain occlusal contact, with a resultant cant in the maxillary occlusal plane and an increase in alveolar height above the inferior dental canal. The face develops a twisted appearance (Figure 25.1B). If abnormal growth is rapid, a lateral open bite may develop on the affected side as the rate of eruption is outpaced by the rate of vertical skeletal growth.

In **hybrid forms** of hemimandibular elongation and hemimandibular hyperplasia, the patients exhibit features of both conditions.

Hemifacial microsomia

Hemifacial microsomia is a congenital disorder, with a prevalence of 1 in 5000 births, that occurs unilaterally in the majority (80%) of cases. The condition is caused by a defect in proliferation and migration of neural crest cells and results in a deficiency of hard and soft tissue structures derived from the **first and second branchial arches**. There is commonly under-development of the temporomandibular joint, mandibular ramus, masticatory muscles and ears on the affected side(s) (Figure 25.1C). In severe cases, the mandibular condyles and ramus may completely fail to develop. Because of reduced vertical growth, there is often under-eruption on the affected side with a resultant **cant** in the maxillary occlusal plane (Figure 25.1C).

Pathological causes

A number of pathological conditions can result in facial asymmetry, but these are out of the scope of this book (readers should refer to textbooks of oral pathology). A rare pathological cause of particular interest to orthodontists is **condylar resorption**. Condylar resorption can occur following traumatic injuries, use of steroids, in connective tissue diseases (e.g. rheumatoid arthritis, scleroderma, systemic lupus erythematosus) and following orthognathic surgery. If one condyle is affected more than the other, there is often a unilateral shift of the chin point to the side of greater resorption. If both condyles are affected, the patient may present with a progressively increasing anterior open bite with or without asymmetry. Treatment should only be considered once the primary pathology has been stabilised and should avoid ramus surgery as there is a risk of re-triggering the primary pathology. Treatment can often be undertaken with genioplasty alone ± maxillary surgery.

Functional causes

A **lateral mandibular displacement**, due to an occlusal interference, can be the cause of a small mandibular dental centreline shift and displacement of the chin point. Treatment in such cases should be directed at removing the occlusal interference (see Chapter 30).

Management of asymmetries

Before treating asymmetries of developmental origin it is important to ensure that the **abnormal growth pattern has ceased**. This can be achieved by comparing serial study models, sequential photographs and three-dimensional soft tissue facial scans. Some clinicians undertake 99m-technetium isotope scans to determine if the condyle is actively growing but the results can be unreliable. Ideally, there should be no change between serial records taken at least 6 months apart.

Imaging techniques used to assess asymmetries include conventional radiographs (dental panoramic tomogram (DPT), lateral/posteroanterior cephalogram), three-dimensional computed tomography, and laser scanning or stereophotogrammetry. A discussion of these is outside the scope of this book.

Treatment planning should involve a **joint orthodontic-orthognathic approach**. Patients with hemifacial microsomia should be managed by dedicated craniofacial teams. Where a developmental asymmetry is identified at a young age (e.g. hemifacial microsomia), a **hybrid functional appliance** can be used to maximise growth on the affected side. Such appliances may create a more favourable environment to encourage growth of the deficient condyle and also help level any maxillary cant by selective molar eruption (Figure 25.1D). This can simplify later surgical treatment but requires considerable compliance.

Patients with severe asymmetries (e.g. hemifacial microsomia) who have aesthetic and functional problems may be treated at a young age (5–8 years) with **distraction osteogenesis** (see Chapter 44) or a **costochondral bone graft** if there is complete absence of a condyle. This is a temporary measure, as the abnormal growth pattern will continue, but finite correction can be undertaken at the end of growth.

In severe cases of hemimandibular elongation and hemimandibular hyperplasia, it may be necessary to consider abolishing the abnormal growth pattern during adolescence. This will involve **condylar shaving** for removing the abnormal cartilaginous growth site. Patients may require surgery later for finite correction.

Finite treatment is undertaken at the end of growth using a comprehensive **orthodontic-orthognathic approach**. After joint planning, orthodontic decompensation is undertaken, followed by surgery to correct the underlying skeletal asymmetry. Surgery will often involve a bilateral sagittal split osteotomy with asymmetric moves ± a Le Fort 1 maxillary procedure to correct any cant in the maxillary occlusal plane.

Often patients with an asymmetry in the chin point will also have asymmetries in other regions of the face (e.g. nose). In such cases it is important while obtaining **informed consent** to make the patient aware that their attention may be diverted towards these issues once the primary focus of their concern, the chin point, has been normalised. It is not possible to make the face totally symmetrical.

Once the underlying skeletal asymmetry has been treated it may be necessary to undertake **secondary surgical procedures** to correct any underlying deficiency/excess. Mild soft tissue deficiencies can be masked by fat transfer (e.g. Coleman fat graft) whereas more major defects may require free flap transfer. In cases of hemimandibular hyperplasia, lower mandibular border recontouring may be necessary to help compensate for excessive vertical growth.

26 Open bite malocclusion

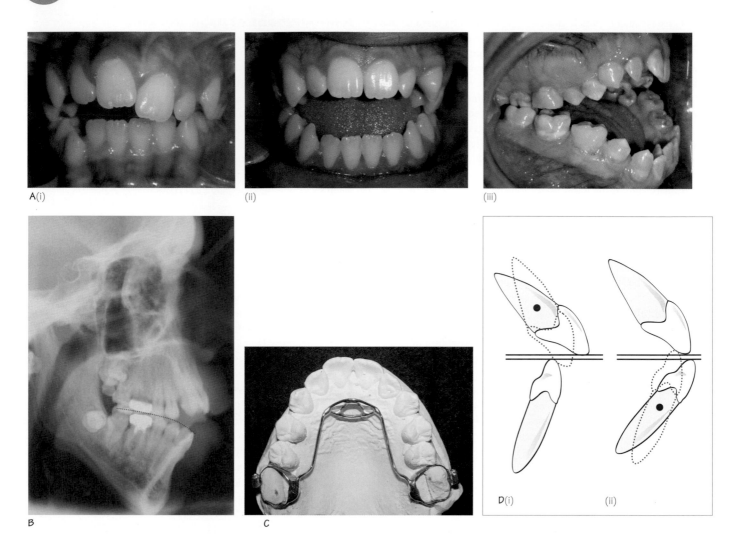

Figure 26.1 (**A**) Examples of open bite: (i) an asymmetrical AOB caused by digit sucking, (ii) a severe symmetrical AOB caused by an increased lower anterior face height and macroglossia and (iii) a severe skeletal AOB extending backwards to produce a posterior open bite. (**B**) A reverse curve of spee in the lower arch is often an indication that the tongue may play an important part in the aetiology of AOB. (**C**) A habit-breaking appliance can be cemented onto the maxillary first permanent molars. It acts as a reminder and makes digit sucking less pleasurable. It should be left *in situ* for a least six months after the habit has stopped. (**D**) Retroclination of the (i) upper and (ii) lower incisors with fixed appliances can help with anterior open bite closure.

An anterior open bite (AOB) exists when there is no vertical overlap between the maxillary and mandibular incisors with the molars in occlusion (Figure 26.1A). The prevalence of AOB shows **ethnic variation** with 2–4% of Caucasians and 5–10% of African Caribbeans being affected. AOB can be classified as mild (1–2 mm), moderate (2–4 mm) or severe (>4 mm), and it may extend posteriorly into the molar region to form a **posterior open bite**. An AOB may also be classified as dental or skeletal, depending on its aetiology, and as symmetrical or asymmetrical depending on its appearance.

Aetiology of AOB

Box 26.1 lists the factors that may contribute to the development of AOB.

Skeletal factors

AOB may be associated with an **increased lower anterior face height**

Box 26.1 Possible aetiological factors in the development of anterior open bite

Skeletal factors
- Increased lower anterior face height
- Condylar resorption

Soft tissue factors
- Forward tongue posture
- Endogenous tongue thrust
- Macroglossia
- Chronic nasal obstruction
- Reduced muscle tone

Habits
- Digit sucking

(LAFH) when the eruptive capacity of the incisors is exceeded. When there is a **clockwise (backward) mandibular growth rotation**, the chances of AOB development are increased. Diagnostic clues to a significant skeletal aetiology include increased LAFH, increased maxillary–mandibular planes angle and a co-existing posterior open bite. An AOB can occur with a skeletal I, II or III pattern.

AOB may develop following **condylar resorption** – a rare condition occurring secondary to mandibular trauma, connective tissue diseases that can affect the temporomandibular joint (e.g. rheumatoid arthritis, systemic sclerosis) and following orthognathic surgery. Resorption of the mandibular condyles results in a reduction in ramus height and clockwise (backwards) rotation of the body of the mandible.

Soft tissue factors

A **forward tongue posture**, where the tongue rests between the incisors, may obstruct incisor eruption (Figure 8.1F). This should not be confused with a *secondary adaptive tongue thrust*, in which the tongue moves forward during swallowing to contact the lips and form an anterior oral seal *secondary* to an AOB. A diagnostic feature on the lateral cephalograph suggesting forward tongue posture is the presence of a reverse curve of Spee in the lower arch caused by reduced incisor eruption (Figure 26.1B). **An endogenous tongue thrust**, characterised by forward thrusting of the tongue on swallowing, is a rare cause of AOB. It may be associated with stigmatism (lisping), incisor proclination and excess contraction of the lips during swallowing.

True **macroglossia** is a rare cause of AOB that may be difficult to diagnose. Suggestive features include a protrusive tongue posture and reverse curve of Spee in the mandibular arch. Patients with **chronic nasal obstruction** (due to adenoidal enlargement) *may* develop AOB malocclusion because a continuous open mouth posture leads to over-eruption of the molars and an increase in LAFH (see Chapter 8). Those with **reduced muscular tone**, as in muscular dystrophy, may be prone to AOB due to excessive vertical facial growth (Figure 26.1Aiii).

Habits

Digit sucking can lead to an **asymmetrical** *dental* AOB which is worst on the side that the digit is sucked (Figure 26.1Ai). Not all digit suckers develop AOB, the important factors being the **duration** and **frequency** of the habit. Those who suck for ≥6 hours a day often develop significant malocclusions. The inserted digit(s) limit incisor eruption, cause upper incisor proclination and act like an anterior bite plane by allowing molar eruption. There is often an associated posterior crossbite (Chapter 30).

Treatment of AOB

There are several approaches for the management of AOB. The presence of an AOB is not an absolute indication for treatment as it may be accepted whilst other aspects of a malocclusion are corrected (e.g. crowding, increased overjet). Mild AOB in the mixed dentition may **resolve spontaneously** because of incisor eruption, favourable skeletal growth and improved lip competency. Possible **benefits of treatment** include:

- Improved ability to incise and chew food.
- Improved aesthetics, especially with orthognathic surgery, due to improved incisor display at rest and during smiling, a reduction in LAFH and improved lip competency.

- Improved speech? There is *no* evidence that AOB correction improves stigmatism (lisping) although patients may demand treatment on this basis.

It is important that **habits** are terminated before commencing orthodontic treatment. **Dummy sucking** (particularly with a deflating 'orthodontic friendly' dummy) is preferable to digit sucking as it is likely to stop by the age of 6 years. Habits persisting following eruption of the permanent incisors should be actively discouraged. This involves patient education and use of reminders such as plasters/gloves on the digits or unpleasant tasting nail polish. If unsuccessful, a **fixed deterrent appliance** (Figure 26.1C) can be used to make the habit less pleasurable. Stopping before establishment of the permanent dentition often results in **spontaneous resolution**, which can be monitored using serial study models over 6–9 months. If habits continue into the permanent dentition, self-correction is less likely and orthodontics can be considered once the habit has ceased.

Orthodontic treatment can be considered where an AOB is mild and treatment is likely to be stable. **Fixed appliances** can be used in Class II (± headgear to limit molar extrusion) or Class III cases to reduce mild AOB principally by uprighting the maxillary incisors in Class II cases and the mandibular incisors in Class III cases (Figure 26.1D). Incisor extrusion for AOB correction is highly **unstable** in skeletal AOB or where the tongue is an important aetiological factor.

There are a number of **removable appliance techniques** incorporating **high pull headgear** for the management of AOB co-existing with Class II malocclusion. These aim to limit molar eruption and posterior vertical maxillary growth thereby encouraging anti-clockwise (forward) rotation of the mandible. Use of headgear also causes maxillary incisor retraction, leading to uprighting, which favours AOB closure. Success depends on excellent patient compliance, with 12–14 hours daily headgear wear, and treatment being undertaken for the duration of the pubertal growth spurt. Headgear should not be used in Class III malocclusion as maxillary restraint will lead to deterioration of a Class III relationship. Some clinicians use the **vertical pull chin cup** in Class III cases to limit excessive vertical and horizontal mandibular growth, however, compliance issues are similar to those with use of headgear and the long-term benefits are unknown.

Active retention (see Chapter 41) following treatment using an upper removable retainer with posterior bite blocks, and headgear in Class II cases, may help to improve treatment stability.

Orthognathic surgery can be used in moderate/severe skeletal AOB after completion of facial growth. Following orthodontic decompensation, surgery will often involve posterior maxillary impaction which will reduce the LAFH. This can be associated with mandibular advancement (Class II) or setback (Class III). **Tongue reduction**, which is rarely indicated, can be considered for correction of macroglossia.

Stability of AOB correction

Relapse of AOB correction can be related to:

- unfavourable vertical skeletal growth especially if associated with a clockwise (backward) mandibular growth rotation;
- a forward tongue posture, macroglossia or a primary endogenous tongue thrust;
- continuation of digit sucking;
- relapse of inappropriately extruded incisors.

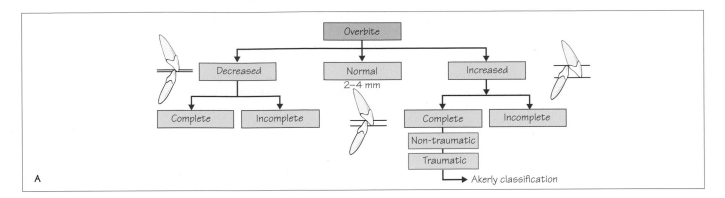

A

Table 27.1 Akerly classification of traumatic overbite.

Akerly 1	The lower incisors occlude with the palatal mucosa causing mucosal trauma away from the patatal gingival margin	
Akerly 2	The lower incisors occlude with and traumatise the palatal gingival margins of the upper incisors	
Akerly 3	Traumatic occlusion leads to stripping of the lower labial and the upper palatal gingivae	
Akerly 4	The incisors sheer past each other causing wear on the palatal aspects of the upper incisors and sometimes the labial aspect of the lower incisors. This may be associated with loss of posterior dental support and/or a parafunctional habit	

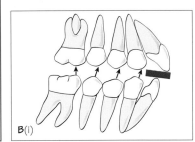

B(i)

Table 27.2 Methods for reducing a deep overbite.

Technique	
Removable appliance	• Anterior bite plane • Headgear • Functional appliances
Fixed appliance	• Fixed orthodontic appliances
Orthognathic surgery	• Mandibular advancement • Lower labial segment setdown
Resorative treatment	• Restoration of the posterior occlusal vertical dimension • Occlusal splints • Dahl appliance

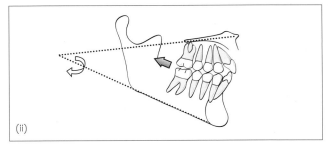

(ii)

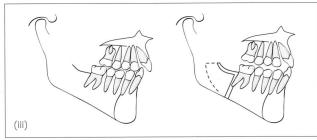

(iii)

Figure 27.1 (**A**) Classification of overbite. (**B**) Methods for reducing a deep overbite. (i) An anterior bite plane encourages molar eruption and prevents incisor eruption. (ii) Distal movement of the maxillary molars results in bite opening by the wedge effect. (iii) In non-growing individuals with Class II deep bite malocclusion, anterior-inferior surgical repositioning of the mandible can reduce the OB and increase the LAFH.

The overbite (OB) is the vertical overlap of the mandibular incisors by the maxillary incisors, measured perpendicular to the occlusal plane, with the posterior teeth in occlusion. The normal OB measures 2–4 mm, that is the upper incisors cover approximately one-third of the crown of the lower incisors. A normal OB is important for incision during mastication and anterior guidance during mandibular excursions. Figure 27.1A shows the **classification** of OB. A complete OB exists when the lower incisors occlude with the upper incisors or the palatal gingiva/mucosa. Soft tissue contact may be traumatic (if there is soreness, gingival inflammation and/or recession) or non-traumatic. An OB may also be traumatic when the upper incisors impinge on the lower labial gingivae and exacerbate periodontal destruction. The Akerly classification is used to categorise deep traumatic OB (Table 27.1).

Aetiology of deep OB

Skeletal factors
The lower incisors will continue to erupt until they make contact with opposing teeth, the palatal mucosa or the resting tongue. When the overjet is increased, as in a **skeletal II pattern**, the lower incisors continue to erupt until they meet palatal tissue. The deep OB is exacerbated by a **reduced lower anterior face height** (LAFH) as the distance that the lower incisors have to erupt to span the height of the intermaxillary space is reduced. An **anti-clockwise (forward) mandibular growth rotation** also favours the development of a deep OB.

Soft tissues factors
A **high lower-lip line** can result in retroclination of the maxillary incisors, which increases the interincisal angle and favours deep OB formation.

Local factors
A poorly formed maxillary central incisor **cingulum** favours overeruption of the lower incisors.

Treatment
Treatment approaches for managing deep OB are summarised in Table 27.2. The **benefits** of reducing deep OB include:
• Elimination of gingival trauma. Plaque control is also essential for treatment success.
• Facilitation of overjet reduction during comprehensive orthodontic treatment.
• Facilitation of restorative treatment.

Orthodontic correction of deep OB is best undertaken in growing individuals as vertical facial growth helps to reduce OB and maintain stable correction. Tooth movements that result in bite opening include:
• upper and lower incisor intrusion;
• upper and lower molar eruption;
• proclination of the upper and lower incisors;
• distal movement of the maxillary molars.

A **flat anterior bite plane** (Figure 27.1Bi), incorporated into an upper removable appliance, prevents lower incisor eruption and encourages lower molar eruption. Eruption of the lower molars reduces the OB by increasing the LAFH and is only stable in growing patients as compensatory vertical mandibular ramus growth is required to prevent re-intrusion. **Functional appliances** work principally by encouraging lower molar eruption and increasing vertical skeletal growth.

Fixed orthodontic appliances can be used to reduce a deep OB by upper or lower incisor intrusion, upper and lower incisor proclination, molar eruption or a combination of these factors. The use of **Class II intermaxillary elastics** encourages lower molar extrusion. Incisor proclination is often undertaken in Class II division 2 malocclusion as the incisors are retroclined. Lower incisor proclination should be undertaken with caution as it is prone to relapse (see Chapter 11). Lower incisor intrusion is often the treatment of choice in non-growing patients because molar extrusion is likely to be unstable. Upper incisor intrusion should be attempted with caution as it will reduce the amount of incisor exposure both at rest and during smiling which may give the face an aged appearance (Figure 6.1F).

Cervical pull headgear (Figure 37.1Di) can result in bite opening by extruding the upper molars. Distal movement of the maxillary molars also contributes to bite opening by hinging open the maxillary-mandibular planes angle (**wedge effect**, Figure 27.1Bii). **J-hook headgear** for upper incisor intrusion is rarely used because of concerns about safety.

Orthognathic surgery can be used in non-growing patients to reduce a deep OB too severe to be corrected by the techniques described above. A commonly performed procedure is the bilateral sagittal split osteotomy with forwards and downwards repositioning of the mandible (Figure 27.1Biii).

Restorative treatment, involving increasing the **posterior occlusal vertical dimension**, can be considered where there is loss of posterior dental support. An **occlusal splint** can be given to bruxists for nocturnal wear to reduce the detrimental effect of parafunctional forces. The **Dahl appliance**, which works by incisor intrusion and molar eruption, can be used for creating sufficient space for the restoration of the palatal surfaces of the maxillary incisors if necessary.

Stability of OB correction
The stability of OB correction depends on a number of factors:
• Correction of the interincisal angle (normally 135°) and ensuring that the lower incisors have a positive occlusal stop on the palatal surface of the maxillary incisors. Achieving these goals involves ensuring that the lower incisor edge is ahead of the upper incisor root centroid. The centroid is the midpoint of the upper incisor root.
• Favourable mandibular growth. OB correction maybe unstable in patients with a significant anti-clockwise (forward) mandibular growth rotation. Vertical mandibular ramus growth is also important for stability following molar extrusion.
• Minimising proclination of the mandibular incisors. If inadequately retained, proclined incisors will often upright following treatment and re-erupt.

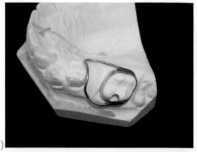

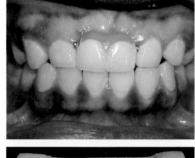

A(i)

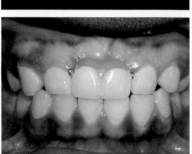

(ii)

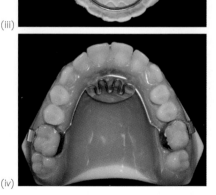

(iii)

(iv)

Table 28.1 *The sequence of classically described serial extractions.*

Procedure	Notes
Extraction of four deciduous canines	Undertaken at the age of approximately 8 years in a child of average dental development, at the time of eruption of the maxillary lateral incisors. This should allow spontaneous alignment of the incisors at the expense of canine space
Extraction of the first deciduous molars	Undertaken at the age of approximately 9 years when the roots of the first premolars are half formed. The aim is to encourage the first premolars to erupt before the canines, which is often not the case in the lower arch
Extraction of the first premolars	Undertaken near the time of eruption of the canines, after confirming that they are buccally palpable and mesially angulated, if there is sufficient crowding to warrant premolar extractions and if all other teeth are present and sound.

Early mixed dentition
Digit sucking habits (Chapter 22) Delayed eruption of the maxillary central incisor (Chapter 31) Supernumerary teeth (Chapter 34) Early loss of deciduous teeth (Chapter 21) Impaction of first permanent molars (Chapter 31) Anterior crossbites (Chapter 30) Posterior crossbites (Chapter 30) Severe crowding (Chapter 21) Increased overjet (Chapter 22)
Late mixed dentition
Ectopic maxillary canines (Chapter 32) Poor-quality first permanent molars (Chapter 29) Infraocclusion Hypodontia (Chapter 33) Traumatic overbites (Chapter 27) Increased overjet (Chapter 22)
Early permanent dentition
Impacted teeth Crowding Hypodontia

Box 28.1 *Interceptive treatment may benefit a number of the clinical situations outlined.*

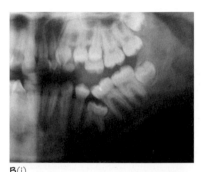

B(i)

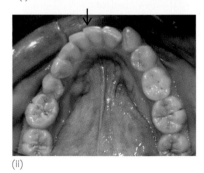

(ii)

Figure 28.1 (**A**) (i) Band and loop space maintainer to retain the second deciduous molar space, (ii) a partial denture used to replace missing central incisors, (iii) a lingual arch used to maintain lower arch length and (iv) a Nance palatal arch. (**B**) (i, ii) A case with total submergence of the lower left second deciduous molar. Note the tipping of the adjacent teeth (i) and significant displacement of the centreline to the left (ii).

Interceptive orthodontics involves the early treatment of occlusal disturbances to eliminate or simplify their future management. Such intervention is usually undertaken during the mixed dentition stage of development. Box 28.1 outlines a number of situations encountered during various stages of the developing dentition that may benefit from interceptive treatment. Many of these are discussed elsewhere in detail and the relevant chapter numbers are given. This chapter will focus on interceptive measures for the management of crowding, space maintenance and infraocclusion.

Serial extractions

Serial extractions were introduced in the 1940s to treat Class I malocclusion complicated by **severe labial segment crowding**. The aim was to spontaneously guide the developing dentition into good alignment without the use of appliance treatment by selectively timing deciduous and permanent tooth extractions. The classic sequence of serial extraction is summarised in Table 28.1. The disadvantages of the procedure include:

• Extractions may require multiple procedures under general anaesthesia and are a stressful experience for the patient.
• Early loss of the first deciduous molar may result in mesial drift of the buccal segments with further space loss.
• The lower canine may still erupt into the first deciduous molar space before the first premolar resulting in first premolar impaction.
• There is no spontaneous correction of an incorrect incisor relationship, hence it is only useful in Class I cases.
• There is a risk of lower incisor retroclination and deepening of the overbite.
• Patients may still require later appliance treatment.

Serial extraction is rarely undertaken in its classically described form because of the disadvantages stated above and the current wide availability of fixed appliances. Occasionally, a modified version of the procedure may be carried out (e.g. extraction of deciduous canines to allow alignment of the incisors or for interceptive treatment of palatal maxillary canines) to simplify later appliance treatment.

Space maintenance

Space maintenance is a useful interceptive procedure aimed to prevent the development of crowding following:

• early loss of deciduous teeth;
• delayed eruption or early loss of permanent maxillary incisors;
• before exfoliation of the second deciduous molars to preserve leeway space for the relief of crowing.

Space maintenance should be considered in a number of situations:
(1) following early loss of the second deciduous molars;
(2) when the first deciduous molars are lost before eruption of the first permanent molars;
(3) following unilateral loss of the deciduous canines.

This is particularly important if more than 3–6 months will elapse before eruption of the permanent successors and if there is adequate space to accommodate these teeth. Early loss of the second deciduous molars results in mesial migration of the first permanent molars and can lead to second premolar impaction. The loss of the first deciduous molars, before eruption of the first permanent molars, may lead to *early* mesial shift of the first permanent molars with loss of space for the first premolars. Early loss of the deciduous canines can result in a centreline shift, retroclination of the incisors and loss of space for the permanent canine.

If there is delayed eruption or early loss of a permanent maxillary central incisor one should consider space maintenance before mesial migration of the lateral incisor. A **partial denture** or upper removable appliance also has the benefit of restoring aesthetics.

A number of space maintaining appliances are available. The **band and loop** (Figure 28.1Ai) is a fixed cantilevered space maintainer consisting of a steel band soldered to a loop that maintains arch length. The band is usually placed on the first permanent molar. This form of space maintainer can only span a single unit of space without the risk of distortion or fracture and is therefore useful in cases of unilateral loss of one deciduous molar. In cases of bilateral loss, or where more than one unit is missing per quadrant, a lingual arch should be considered. Disadvantages of the band and loop space maintainer include the risk of decalcification and overeruption of teeth opposite the loop.

As this appliance is fixed it does not depend on patient compliance for insertion.

Partial dentures and upper removable appliances are useful when multiple units are missing, including maxillary incisors (Figure 28.1Aii). The main advantages of their use is that they may restore aesthetics and function and prevent overeruption. A major disadvantage is the dependence on patient compliance for insertion.

A **distal shoe** is a banded custom-made appliance designed to prevent mesial movement of unerupted first permanent molars following early loss of second deciduous molars. The appliance is similar in appearance to the band and loop but has a gingival extension at the end of the loop that extends subgingivally 1 mm below the mesial marginal ridge of the first permanent molar. A removable acrylic version of this appliance can be constructed if both the first and second deciduous molars are lost prematurely.

A **lingual arch** (Figure 28.1Aiii) is indicated when there is bilateral loss of lower deciduous molars. This appliance is banded onto the first permanent molars and extends anteriorly to contact the lingual surface of the incisors. It essentially maintains arch length by preventing mesial drift of the first molars and retroclination of the incisors.

The **Nance palatal arch** (Figure 28.1Aiv) is the equivalent of a lingual arch used in the upper arch. Instead of contacting the palatal surface of the incisors anteriorly, an acrylic button contacts the palate. This appliance prevents rotation and mesial tipping of the first permanent molars following early loss of the maxillary deciduous molars. The Nance palatal and lingual arches can be used to preserve Leeway space if placed before exfoliation of the deciduous molars in cases of mild crowding when a non-extraction approach is planned.

Infraocclusion

Infraocclusion is a consequence of ankylosis – the anatomical fusion between cementum and alveolar bone. Ankylosis limits the compensatory eruptive mechanism that maintains the level of the occlusal plane during vertical skeletal development. The prevalence of infraocclusion is reported to be between 1% and 9% with the mandibular first and second deciduous molars being most commonly affected. It is more common among relatives which suggests a genetic predisposition.

The potential occlusal consequences of infraocclusion are summarised in Table 9.2 and illustrated in Figure 28.1B. Consequences such as tipping of adjacent teeth and centreline shift occur as a consequence of tension arising within the transseptal fibres that interconnect adjacent teeth (Figure 9.1A).

The management of infraocclusion of deciduous molars depends on whether the permanent successor is present or absent. If present, eruption of the permanent successor will be delayed by an average of 6 months. The occlusion should be monitored unless there is severe tipping of adjacent teeth with space loss, in which case extraction of the submerging molar (± space maintenance) should be considered.

When infraocclusion affects a deciduous molar with no permanent successor, the rate of progression may be slow and depend on the rate of remaining vertical skeletal growth. Treatment options include:

• **Monitoring** – if infraocclusion is mild and there have been no occlusal disturbances.
• **Restoration** – of the occlusal surface to help prevent tipping of adjacent teeth and over-eruption of opposing teeth.
• **Extraction** – if adjacent teeth are tipped and if there is a risk of total submergence.

Figure 29.1 (**A**) Timing of the extraction of mandibular first permanent molars.

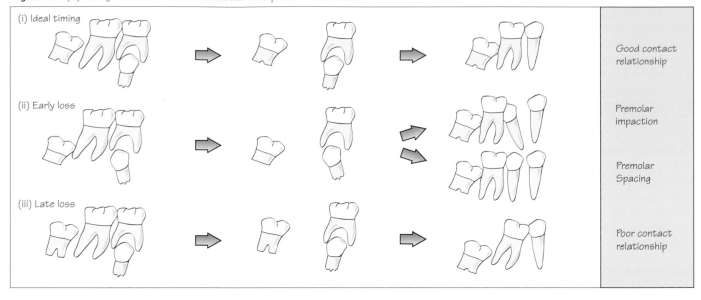

(i) Ideal timing — Good contact relationship

(ii) Early loss — Premolar impaction — Premolar Spacing

(iii) Late loss — Poor contact relationship

Figure 29.1 (**B**) Cases later requiring space for relief of crowding or overjet correction.

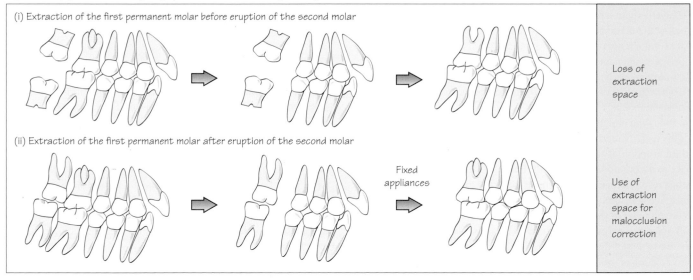

(i) Extraction of the first permanent molar before eruption of the second molar — Loss of extraction space

(ii) Extraction of the first permanent molar after eruption of the second molar — Fixed appliances — Use of extraction space for malocclusion correction

Figure 29.1 (**C**) Compensating extractions.

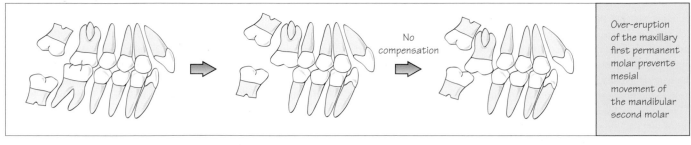

No compensation — Over-eruption of the maxillary first permanent molar prevents mesial movement of the mandibular second molar

The first permanent molars are considered to be the most caries-prone teeth in the permanent dentition probably because of their early eruption and exposure to the oral environment. These teeth can also be affected by hypomineralisation/hypoplasia and may be ankylosed in rare cases.

During the mixed dentition stage of dental development, general dentists and orthodontists may encounter patients with poor prognosis first permanent molars. In this situation, extraction of the teeth and space closure or use of the extraction space for future orthodontic treatment should be considered. This chapter provides guidelines about treatment planning for patients in the mixed dentition stage, who have first molars with a poor prognosis.

Consequences of loss of mandibular first permanent molars

Ideal timing (Figure 29.1Ai)
The ideal developmental stage for enforced loss of first permanent molars is when the furcation of the second permanent molar is just beginning to form which normally corresponds to a chronological age of 8–9 years. Loss at this stage usually results in satisfactory spontaneous space closure and the establishment of a good contact point relationship between the second molar and second premolar. There will be some spontaneous resolution of premolar crowding and the third molars will almost certainly erupt if they are present.

Early loss (Figure 29.1Aii)
Extraction before the age of 8 years often results in significant distal migration of the second premolar which may then become impacted against the second molar. This migration occurs because the second premolar lies in an unrestrained position apical to the roots of the second deciduous molar and the extraction socket of the first permanent molars provides an easy path to eruption.

Late loss (Figure 29.1Aiii)
If the first permanent molar is extracted during or after eruption of the second molar, space closure will be poor, and there will be significant mesial tipping and lingual rolling of the second molar.

Consequences of loss of maxillary first permanent molars
The timing of extractions in the maxilla is less critical than in the mandible because the second permanent molar develops with a distal angulation. The advantage of this is that the root is already in a good position and it is just a case of the second molar crown moving mesially to establish a good relationship. The first permanent molar may be extracted even when the second molar is about to erupt to achieve a satisfactory result. Timing in the mandible is much more critical as the second molar often develops with a mesial angulation and the alveolar bone is more dense.

Factors to consider when planning the loss of first permanent molars

Restorative state of the first permanent molar
Consideration should be given to the extraction of teeth with large restorations, pulpal necrosis or severe hypoplasia.

Presence of crowding
Loss of the first permanent molars is likely to result in spontaneous resolution of crowding in the premolar region. However, if there is significant crowding in the labial segment, consideration may be given to keeping the first permanent molar until the second molar erupts, and using the first permanent molar extraction space for the relief of crowding in combination with fixed appliance therapy (Figure 29.1B). If, however, the first permanent molar has an extremely poor prognosis and must be extracted, space for the relief of crowding and/or overjet reduction can be obtained later by premolar extractions, use of headgear to distalise the maxillary buccal segments or functional appliances for overjet correction.

All attempts should be made to conserve the first permanent molars in arches with spacing because space closure is likely to be poor with the added loss of these teeth.

Occlusal relationship
In Class I cases with labial segment crowding, extraction of the first permanent molar may be considered once the second molar has erupted to use the extraction space to resolve the crowding (Figure 29.1Bii).

In Class II cases space is required to correct the incisal relationship and for the relief of crowding. An attempt should be made to preserve the first permanent molar until the second molar erupts, to use the space.

In Class III cases, the first permanent molar may be required to provide retention for removable appliance treatment and it may be important for anchorage in the lower arch for incisor retraction.

In all the instances described above, **specialist orthodontic advice** is recommended before the extraction of first permanent molars.

Position of the second premolar
If the second premolar lies below the roots of the second deciduous molar and is distally angulated, it may erupt distally into the first permanent molar socket as this provides the path of least resistance to eruption. The second deciduous molar should be extracted at the same time as the first permanent molar in such cases to encourage a normal path of second premolar eruption.

Balancing and compensating extractions
Balancing is extraction of a contralateral tooth, which need not be the first permanent molar, to prevent shifting of the dental centreline in **crowded** cases. Consideration should be given to balancing the loss of a first permanent molar to preserve the centreline with teeth other than the contralateral first permanent molar if they have a poorer long-term prognosis.

Compensating is the extraction of the opposing molar to prevent its overeruption. When a **mandibular** first permanent molar is lost, over-eruption of the maxillary first permanent molar can prevent mesial migration of the mandibular second molar and therefore compensation should be considered (Figure 29.1C). When the **maxillary** first permanent molar is lost, the mandibular first permanent molar does not tend to over-erupt, hence compensation is not necessary when extracting the maxillary first permanent molar. Balancing and compensating extractions are only indicated during the mixed dentition stage, and not in the permanent dentition, because spontaneous tooth movement occurs more readily as the dentition is establishing itself than once it is established.

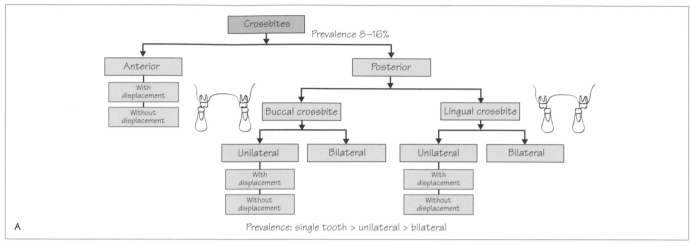

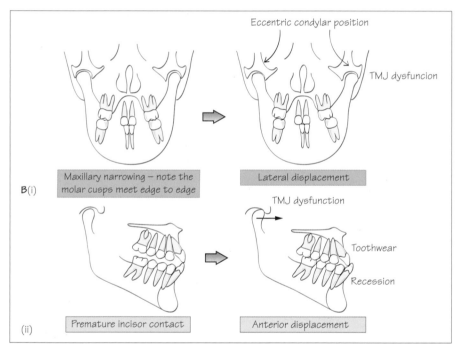

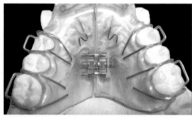

C(i)
An upper removable appliance with a midline screw can be used for posterior crossbite correction. The screw is turned a quarter turn a week producing 0.25 mm/wk expansion.

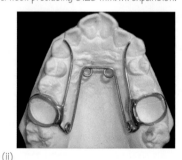

(ii)
The Quad helix appliance for correcting posterior crossbite. The appliance is fixed and can also act as a habit breaker.

◄ An upper removable appliance with a Z-spring can be used for anterior crossbite correction. Molar acrylic capping can be used if the freeway space is inadequate to allow the incisors to cross the bite.

Rapid maxillary expansion can be used before ▶ closure of the mid-palatal suture which occurs at approx 17–18 years. The screw is turned twice daily to produce 0.5 mm expansion/day. Retention is important to maintain correction.

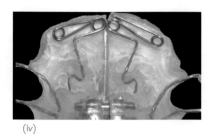

(iv)

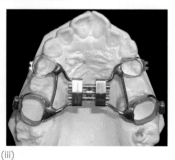

(iii)

Figure 30.1 (**A**) Classification of crossbites. (**B**) Crossbites with mandibular displacement: (i) posterior crossbite and (ii) anterior crossbite. (**C**) Fixed and removable appliance techniques for correction of crossbites.

A crossbite can be defined as an abnormal relationship between opposing teeth in a buccopalatal or labiopalatal direction. It is a common malocclusion affecting between **8% and 16%** of the population. Figure 30.1A gives a classification of crossbites. An anterior crossbite exists when one or more of the maxillary incisors occlude lingual to the lower incisors with the posterior teeth in occlusion. A posterior buccal crossbite occurs when the buccal cusps of the lower molars occlude buccal to the fossae of the upper molars. A lingual crossbite (also termed a scissor bite) exists when the buccal cusps of the lower molars occlude lingual to the fossae of the upper molars. It is important that patients presenting with crossbites are examined for a mandibular displacement.

Aetiology of crossbites

Skeletal factors
A **narrow maxilla** can result in a unilateral or bilateral buccal crossbite. A unilateral crossbite most commonly arises when there is symmetrical narrowing of the maxilla to the extent that the upper and lower molar cusps meet tip to tip. This produces a **mandibular displacement** to one side to improve intercuspation leaving a crossbite on the side to which the mandible displaces (Figure 30.1B). When the maxilla is repositioned relative to the mandible (**skeletal III pattern**) there may be an anterior crossbite or a *relative* buccal crossbite because a narrower part of the maxilla opposes a wider part of the mandible (Figure 8.1C). When the mandible is retropositioned relative to the maxilla (**skeletal II pattern**) a lingual crossbite may occur in the buccal segments. Significant **asymmetrical mandibular growth** is a rare cause of unilateral buccal crossbite (see Chapter 25).

Habits and soft tissue factors
When a **thumb or finger sucking** habit is of adequate duration and intensity a unilateral buccal crossbite may result. This occurs because the balance of soft tissue forces, with downward displacement of the tongue and increased pressure from the cheeks, favours contraction of the maxillary arch. Patients with **chronic nasal obstruction** may also develop crossbites due to narrowing of the maxilla. Mouth breathing leads to depression of the tongue from its normal resting position in the palate, which alters the balance of forces between the tongue and cheeks, and favours maxillary narrowing.

Local factors
Dental crowding can lead to the eruption of a tooth into a crossbite relationship. Situations where this is encountered include palatally erupted maxillary lateral incisors and lingually or palatally erupted second premolar teeth associated with early loss of second deciduous molars.

Treatment of crossbites
Benefits of treatment include:
• Elimination of: mandibular displacement, which can lead to temporomandibular joint dysfunction in a susceptible patient; attrition at the site of premature contact; exacerbation of plaque-related recession labial to the lower incisors (anterior crossbite); and perpetuation of a buccal segment crossbite from the mixed dentition into the permanent dentition.

• Space creation for the relief of crowding due to an increase in arch circumference.
• Improvement in smile aesthetics by broadening the smile and reducing buccal corridor width (see Chapter 17).

Anterior crossbite
Anterior crossbites, involving one or two incisors, can be treated using **upper removable appliances** during the mixed dentition. **Fixed appliances** are often employed during the permanent dentition if bodily tooth movement is required and if the crossbite is too severe to be treated by upper incisor proclination alone but also requires retraction of the lower incisors (moderate Class III malocclusion). For correction to be successful there should be a good post-treatment overbite for stability. Care should be taken to ensure that the maxillary canine is not developing labially to a palatally displaced lateral incisor when attempting crossbite correction as labial movement may cause damage to the lateral incisor root. The management of Class III malocclusion is considered in Chapter 24.

Posterior crossbite
The elimination of a **digit-sucking habit** is important before attempting crossbite correction to help maintain stability.

Crossbites in the deciduous or mixed dentition may result from premature contact between the deciduous canines with a resultant lateral mandibular displacement. These maybe treated by **grinding the canines tips** (just the enamel) to eliminate the premature contact.

Before attempting active appliance treatment to correct a buccal segment crossbite, it is important to ensure that the maxillary molars are not already excessively buccally inclined as further tipping maybe unstable and damage their periodontal attachment. **Bilateral buccal crossbites** should be treated with extreme caution. If correction is only partial, or if there is relapse following treatment, there is a risk of creating a unilateral crossbite associated with a mandibular displacement.

A number of removable and fixed appliance techniques are available for the correction of crossbites (Figure 30.1C). The choice of technique is dependent on the type of tooth movement required, the necessity for skeletal expansion and the experience of the operator. **Removable appliances** with a midline expansion screw, the **quad-helix appliance** and **fixed appliances** largely produce expansion by buccal molar tipping. Fifty per cent of expansion produced by **rapid maxillary expansion** is skeletal in origin due to separation at the midpalatal suture. With increasing age, the suture becomes more interlocked such that separation becomes less probable after the age of 17–18 years and should not be attempted. The **functional regulator** functional appliances produce expansion using a buccal shield (Figure 39.1Di) that alters the position of soft tissue balance of the molars towards the cheeks.

In those cases in which there is severe narrowing of the maxillary arch, the only successful method of treatment may be the use of fixed appliances in association with **orthognathic surgery** for maxillary widening.

Stability of crossbite correction
The stability of crossbite correction largely depends on:
• an adequate post-treatment overbite (anterior crossbites);
• not excessively tipping the teeth to achieve correction;
• good posterior intercuspation;
• favourable anteroposterior and transverse skeletal growth.

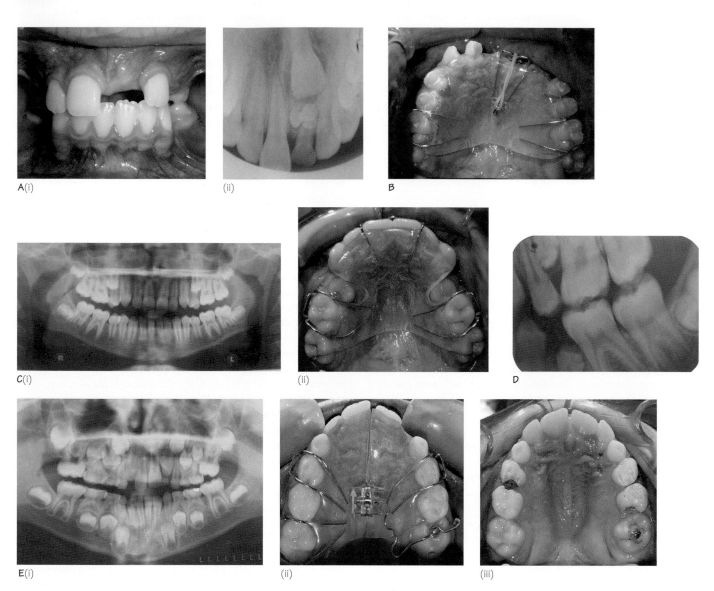

Figure 31.1 (**A**) (i) An asymmetrical pattern of central incisor eruption and eruption of the lateral incisors before a central incisor indicates a problem with central incisor eruption. (ii) Further investigation shows that the upper left central incisor has been prevented from erupting by multiple supernumerary teeth. (**B**) (i) An example of an upper removable appliance (URA) being used to align impacted central incisors. The incisors have been exposed and bonded with a gold chain. Elastic traction is applied to the unerupted teeth from the URA via the gold chain. (**C**) (i) Early loss of second deciduous molars has resulted in maxillary second premolar impaction. (ii) Extraction of the first premolars, followed by space maintenance with a URA has resulted in the eruption of the second premolars into a good position. Surgical removal of the second premolars has been avoided. (**D**) The first premolars should only be extracted to create space if the second premolars are of normal form. In this case, radiographic examination revealed that the crowns of the second premolars were hypoplastic. The second premolars should be extracted in such cases. (**E**) (i) The upper left first permanent molar (UL6) is impacted and causing root resorption of the upper left second deciduous molar. (ii) URA used to apply a distalising force via an occlusal button bonded onto UL6. (iii) Following correction of UL6.

Impaction can be defined as the failure of a tooth to erupt, usually due to crowding or an obstruction (e.g. supernumerary tooth, fibrous tissue). Rarely a tooth may fail to erupt due to failure in the eruptive mechanism (primary failure of eruption, Chapter 9). Some medical conditions (e.g. cleidocranial dysplasia, Table 13.4iii) can be associated with multiple impactions. The aim of this chapter is to give a brief overview of impacted teeth. Chapter 32 focuses on maxillary canine impaction.

Impacted maxillary central incisors

The **prevalence** of impacted maxillary central incisors is reported to be **0.13%**. The most common aetiological factor is the presence of supernumerary teeth but other factors such as trauma (e.g. dilaceration), retention of primary incisors and impaction against fibrous tissue may be important. Impaction should be suspected if the contralateral incisor has erupted more than six months previously or if the lateral incisors have erupted before the central incisors (Figure 31.1A). In such cases a radiographic assessment using an upper anterior occlusal or periapical view(s) is recommended.

The first principle of management is to ensure that **adequate space** is present to accommodate the impacted tooth (9 mm for an average incisor). This may involve extraction of retained deciduous teeth. Secondly, any cause of **obstruction** should be removed. Tuberculate supernumeraries are more commonly associated with incisor impaction than conically shaped teeth (see Chapter 34). In up to 75% of cases, the impacted incisor may erupt spontaneously within 16 months of removal of the supernumerary. Spontaneous improvement is more likely to occur in younger patients with open root apices. **Space maintenance** is important whilst awaiting incisor eruption. If there is no spontaneous improvement one should consider **exposing and bonding** the impacted teeth in order to apply orthodontic traction. As up to 50% of patients may eventually require exposure and bonding, some clinicians perform this procedure at the time of supernumerary removal to eliminate the need for re-operation. It is important for future periodontal health that teeth erupt through **attached gingivae**, which can be achieved either with an apically repositioned flap (for teeth in a low position) or the closed eruption technique (highly placed teeth). A removable appliance can be used to apply traction forces with the advantage of providing good **vertical anchorage** from the palatal vault (Figure 31.1B).

Dilaceration (see Glossary) is often the result of an episode of trauma that disrupts root development. Impacted dilacerated incisors can be aligned following exposure and bonding and application of orthodontic traction. Elective root canal treatment and/or apicectomy may be required if the root apex fenestrates the cortical plate during alignment because of the abnormal root angle. In cases of severe dilaceration, surgical removal may be the only option.

Impacted premolars

Second premolar impaction is most commonly due to early loss of the second deciduous molar(s) and consequent space loss by mesial migration of the first permanent molar. The earlier the tooth is lost, the more space loss is likely to occur, and the greater the crowding. Even in some cases of complete space loss, the second premolars may erupt palatally or lingually. In cases where the second premolar remains unerupted, consideration can be given to **extraction** of the first premolar, **space maintenance**, and awaiting spontaneous eruption of the impacted tooth (Figure 31.1C). This eliminates the need for complex surgical extractions which carry the risk of root and mental nerve damage in the lower arch. There is a small risk that the second premolar may not erupt spontaneously or of space loss if compliance with space maintenance is poor. It is also important to radiographically assess whether the crown of the second premolar is normally formed before making this extraction decision (Figure 31.1D).

If the second premolar(s) are impacted and the arches are otherwise well aligned, consideration can be given to removal of the second permanent molar(s) as this can provide space by spontaneous distal movement of the first permanent molar(s). A specialist orthodontic opinion should be obtained before making any extraction decision.

Impacted first permanent molars

The **prevalence** of first permanent molar impaction is reported to be between **0.75% and 6%**, and it is more common in males than females. The maxillary molar is affected more often than its mandibular counterpart. The prevalence in patients with cleft lip and palate has been reported to be as high as 22%. The aetiology of impaction includes factors such as crowding, ectopic positioning of the first molar crypt and an unfavourable second deciduous molar crown morphology.

Clinically and radiographically the mesial aspect of the first permanent molar becomes impacted beneath the distal bulbosity of the second deciduous molar (Figure 31.1Ei). The severity of the impaction varies with severe cases displaying significant **root resorption** of the deciduous molar with loss of vitality. The complications of impaction include resorption of the deciduous molar root with loss of vitality, space loss and caries of the first permanent molar due to reduced access for cleaning.

A number of **treatment approaches** have been described for impacted first molars including:

* observation;
* separation;
* upper removable appliance or headgear for distal movement;
* fixed appliances;
* extraction of the second deciduous molar.

A period of **observation** should be considered in cases of mild impaction with minimal (<1.5 mm) resorption of the second deciduous molar root. A large proportion of these molars will self-correct. If there is no spontaneous improvement within three to six months, consideration should be given to active treatment.

A brass wire **separator** can be used to attempt to move the first molar distally if there is >1.5 mm of resorption of the second deciduous molar or if no improvement has occurred following observation. The brass wire is inserted around the mesial first molar contact area and should be tightened once a week to produce an adequate disimpacting force.

A distalising force can be applied to the first permanent molar to produce disimpaction with **removable appliances** (Figure 31.1Eii, iii), **fixed appliances** (e.g. a modified transpalatal arch) or **headgear**. Advantages of fixed over removable appliances are that wear is not dependent on patient compliance.

Extraction of the second deciduous molar should be considered as a final option if root resorption is severe as it is likely to lead to space loss and future crowding in the second premolar region.

Impacted third permanent molars

The **prevalence** of third molar impaction is estimated to be **30–50%**, with the mandibular molars being more commonly affected than their maxillary counterparts. The aetiology of impaction is most commonly crowding or an ectopic crypt position. There is a reduced risk of third molar impaction in patients undergoing orthodontic treatment involving extractions in whom some closure of the extraction space is achieved by mesial molar movement. This can be stated to patients as an advantage of extraction treatment, however, it does not guarantee successful eruption and should not be a primary reason for recommending extractions.

Complications associated with impacted third molars include dental caries, pericoronitis, cyst formation and damage to the second molar. There is no evidence that third molar impaction results in **late lower incisor crowding**.

Third molars should only be removed if there is associated pathology. If this is not the case, the risks of removal outweigh any benefits. The risks of removal include inferior alveolar and lingual nerve damage, infection and the risks inherent in general anaesthesia. If an impaction is mild and the tooth is partially erupted, a fixed appliance may be considered for alignment.

32 Impacted maxillary canines

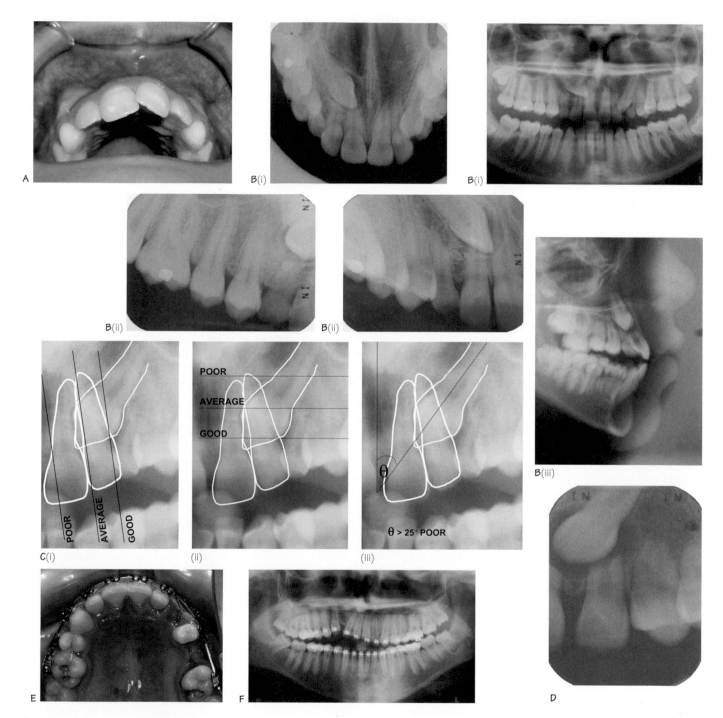

Figure 32.1 (**A**) The canines should be palpable buccally by the age of 10 years. Note the canine bulge in the figure. If the canines are not palpable, one should consider radiographic examination to determine their position. (**B**) Radiographic localisation of impacted maxillary canines. (i) Vertical parallax using a DPT and upper anterior occlusal radiograph. Note that the canine moves in the direction of the tube shift indicating a palatal position. (ii) Horizontal parallax using two periapical views taken at different angles. Note the canine moves in the direction of the tube shift. (iii) A lateral cephalogram can also be used to determine the anteroposterior and vertical position of an impacted canine. (**C**) Assessment of the prognosis for canine alignment. (i) The anteroposterior (AP) position can be assessed by drawing a line mesial to the central and lateral incisor and distal to the lateral incisor. The position of the canine crown in relation to these lines indicates the prognosis for alignment in the AP plane. (ii) The vertical position can be assessed by dividing the lateral incisor root into thirds. The position of the canine crown in relation to these lines indicates the prognosis for alignment in the vertical plane. (iii) The angulation of the long axis of the canine can be measured in relationship to a vertical line. An angulation of >25° indicates likely difficulty with alignment. (**D**) The incisor roots are at risk of resorption in the presence of palatally ectopic canines. In this example, both the central and lateral incisor roots were resorbed. (**E**) Alignment of an impacted maxillary left canine using a fixed appliance. The canine has been exposed and bonded and an archwire is being used to apply orthodontic traction. (**F**) The upper right maxillary canine has become ankylosed and has failed to align following the application of orthodontic forces. Note how the adjacent teeth have intruded in response to the orthodontic forces.

Following the third molars, the maxillary canine is the most commonly impacted tooth. The **prevalence** of maxillary canine impaction is **1–2%** with a female:male ratio of 2:1. Eighty-five per cent of impactions are palatal whilst the remainder (15%) occur buccally.

Normal development of the maxillary canine

The maxillary canine begins its development high in the maxilla at the age of 4–5 months. The tooth has a long path of eruption, passing along the distal root surface of the lateral incisor, buccal to the deciduous canine to its final position with eruption at 11–12 years. The canine should be **palpable** high in the buccal sulcus by the age of **10 years** (Figure 32.1A).

Aetiology of canine impaction

• The **genetic theory** states genetic factors may be important in determining crypt position or the direction of eruption.
• The **guidance theory** suggests the distal root surface of the maxillary lateral incisor is important in guiding the maxillary canine into the arch. When the lateral incisor is small or absent there is a predisposition to canine impaction. Nearly 6% of patients with impacted canines have small lateral incisors.
• **Crowding** is the most common cause of buccal canine impaction.

Clinical and radiographic signs of impaction

Clinical signs of impaction include:
• failure to palpate the canine buccally by 10 years of age;
• immobility of the deciduous canine;
• a palatal bulge indicating the presence of the underlying canine;
• inadequate space within the dental arch for canine eruption;
• increased mobility or non-vitality (indicating advanced root resorption) of the maxillary central and lateral incisors
   Radiographic signs include:
• a palatal canine position demonstrated using the parallax technique;
• the canine overlapping the lateral or central incisor root;
• the long axis of the canine angled more than 25° to the vertical plane.

Radiographic assessment of canine position

This is commonly accomplished using the vertical (dental panoramic tomogram (DPT) and upper anterior occlusal radiograph) or horizontal (two periapicals taken at different angles) parallax techniques (Figure 32.1Bi, ii). A palatally positioned canine will move in the same direction as the tube shift between the radiographs. A buccal canine will move in the opposite direction of the tube shift. (Remember SLOB: Same=Lingual; Opposite=Buccal.) A canine in the line of the arch will remain static between tube shifts. A lateral cephalogram can also be used to assess vertical and anteroposterior position (Figure 32.1Bii). Factors to consider when assessing canine position and the prognosis for alignment include the vertical position, horizontal position and angulation (Figure 32.1C).

Management of palatally displaced canines

There are several options for the management of palatally impacted canines:

• extraction of the deciduous canine;
• no treatment;
• orthodontic alignment;
• surgical removal;
• autotransplantation.

Extraction of the deciduous canine in patients aged between **10 and 13 years**, where the permanent canine is palatal, may help to normalise its eruptive path particularly if there is adequate space within the arch. If there is crowding, the chances of normalisation are reduced. If there is no sign of radiographic improvement after 12 months, it is unlikely to occur and other options should be considered.

No treatment is indicated when the patient is poorly motivated. They should be warned about the potential risk of resorption of the adjacent incisor roots (Figure 32.1D) and cystic change within the canine follicle. Annual radiographic review is advised to check for complications.

Orthodontic alignment, following surgical exposure, is indicated in well-motivated patients where the canine has a favourable position. Alignment is most commonly accomplished using fixed appliances with traction applied via a gold chain bonded to the crown of the canine at the time of surgical exposure or to a bracket directly attached to its surface (Figure 32.1E). Space must be available within the arch to accommodate the impacted tooth. This can be gained by redistributing space already present, the use of headgear to distalise the buccal segments or by extractions. Treatment may take between 2 and 2.5 years. Long-term retention may be necessary to maintain the corrected canine position. Very rarely the canine may be ankylosed and fail to align with orthodontic forces (Figure 32.1F). The only option in such cases may be surgical removal.

Surgical removal should be considered when the canine is in a very unfavourable position, in poorly motivated patients in whom orthodontic treatment is contraindicated and in cases of severe crowding. In the latter case the first premolar can be substituted as a canine.

Autotransplantation is defined as the insertion of a tooth, or developing tooth germ, from one site to a surgically created socket within the same individual. This option maybe considered when the canine has an unfavourable position and there is adequate space within the arch to accommodate the tooth. To avoid ankylosis it is important that the periodontal ligament is not damaged during surgical removal and a period of non-rigid fixation is employed following reimplantation. Transplanted teeth which have a mature apex should be root filled within a week. Teeth with incompletely formed roots have a chance of pulpal revascularisation.

Buccally displaced maxillary canines

These represent **15%** of maxillary canine impactions. The most common cause is severe crowing where the canine gets deflected buccally. The canine will erupt in the majority of cases if the crowding is relieved. Sometimes the canine will not erupt even with the provision of space and consideration should be given to surgical exposure (apically repositioned flap or closed eruption technique) followed by orthodontic alignment. If the canine is totally excluded from the dental arch, and the lateral incisor and first premolar have a good contact relationship, consideration should be given to removal of the canine. This option is particularly attractive in poorly motivated individuals.

33 Hypodontia

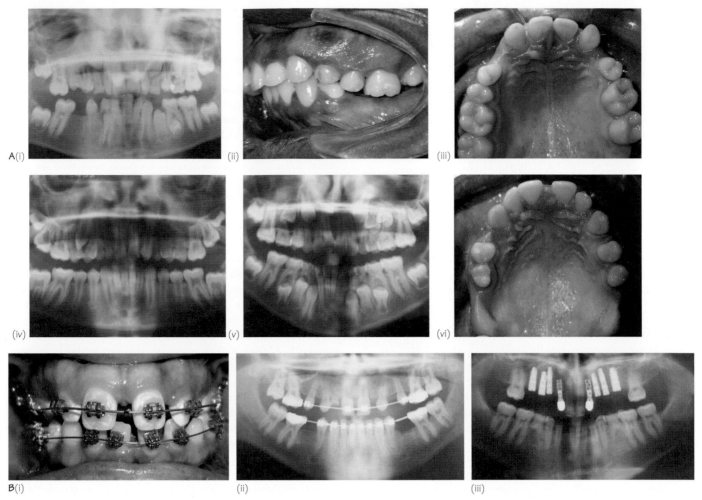

Figure 33.1 (**A**) Features associated with hypodontia include (i) delayed dental development (LL5), (ii) over-eruption of teeth opposing edentulous spaces, (iii) severely rotated premolars, (iv) transposition (between upper right canine and first premolar), (v) taurodontism (upper first permanent molars) and (vi) alveolar atrophy (upper molar spaces). (**B**) The management of hypodontia: (i) fixed appliances can be used for space opening, closing and root paralleling. (ii) Radiographs should be taken before debond to ensure that roots are parallel (note root divergence between the upper first premolars and first molars). (iii) An example of a case restored with implant-retained prosthesis. Implants should only be placed at the end of growth or they will submerge.

Hypodontia is the term used to describe the developmental absence of one or more primary or secondary teeth, excluding third molars. The third molars are excluded as they are commonly missing to varying degrees in 20–25% of people. Hypodontia can be associated with a number of dental anomalies and some medical conditions. It may be classified, according to its severity as:

- **Mild** (1–2 missing teeth)
- **Moderate** (3–5 missing teeth)
- **Severe** (≥6 missing teeth)

More than 80% have mild, ≤10% moderate and ≤1% severe hypodontia. The **prevalence** of hypodontia in the **primary dentition** is **0.3–0.9%** with the maxillary and mandibular lateral incisors being most commonly missing. The absence of a deciduous tooth increases the likelihood of the permanent successor also being absent. The prevalence of hypodontia in the **permanent dentition** is between **3.5% and 6.5%**. Ethnic variation exists, with the common missing tooth types in Caucasians being lower second premolars > upper lateral incisors > upper second premolars > lower central incisors. In some Asian populations, the lower central incisors are reported to be most commonly missing. Overall, females are more commonly affected by hypodontia than males (F:M = 3:2).

Aetiology of hypodontia

The aetiology of hypodontia is multifactorial with both genetic and environmental influences. **Genetics** is important as there is often a family history of hypodontia. An example of an **environmental** factor is the absence of a maxillary lateral incisor associated with a cleft palate where the cleft causes a localised disruption of the dental lamina.

Oral anomalies associated with hypodontia

Features often associated with hypodontia include:
- A **skeletal III pattern**, due to a retrusive maxilla, and a **reduced lower anterior face height (LAFH)**. The likelihood of this increases with the severity of hypodontia.
- **Delayed dental development**. The second premolars are particularly prone to delays in dental development (Figure 33.1Ai) and may not be visible radiographically until the age of 9 years. Hence, a diagnosis of their absence should be made with caution before this age.
- **Microdontia**. This may be localised or generalised and its severity is often correlated with the severity of hypodontia. A common example of microdontia is diminutive or peg-shaped lateral incisors (Figure 16.1Ci).
- **Maxillary canine impaction**. Impaction is associated with the absence, or the presence of a diminutive, maxillary lateral incisor. The root of the lateral incisor may be important in guiding the canine into position (Guidance theory, see Chapter 32). Up to 25% of those with absent lateral incisors may be affected by maxillary canine impaction.
- **Abnormal tooth position**. It is common for permanent teeth to migrate into any spacing present, for over-eruption of teeth opposing edentulous spaces (Figure 33.1Aii), and for teeth to be severely rotated (Figure 33.1Aiii).
- **Transposition** between the maxillary canine and first premolars (Figure 33.1Aiv).
- **Taurodontism**, which is a developmental anomaly where the roots of the molars are shortened at the expense of an elongated pulp chamber. This gives the tooth a classic radiographic appearance (Figure 33.1Av). The roots of taurodont teeth are more prone to orthodontically related root resorption and they offer less anchorage because of their reduced surface area. In addition, endodontic treatment and extractions may be complicated by the abnormal root morphology.
- **Alveolar atrophy**. When a permanent tooth is absent and the deciduous tooth is lost, there will be localised alveolar atrophy which can complicate orthodontic space closure or later implant therapy (Figure 33.1Avi).

Medical conditions associated with hypodontia

The **ectodermal dysplasias** are commonly associated with varying degrees of hypodontia or anodontia (complete absence of teeth). These are a group of genetically transmitted conditions in which there is a defect in the ectodermal tissues. Apart from hypodontia or anodontia, clinical features include hypohidrosis (failure to sweat leading to heat intolerance and dry erythematous skin), hypotrichosis (sparse hair), nail defects and xerostomia. Other medical conditions associated with hypodontia include **Down syndrome**, **cleft lip and palate** and **Hemifacial microsomia**.

Management of hypodontia

The management of hypodontia involves a **multidisciplinary team approach** involving the general dental practitioner, orthodontist, paediatric dentist, prosthodontist and oral surgeon. Treatment depends on the stage of development, the severity of hypodontia and the patient's motivation for treatment. In the majority of patients treatment is undertaken because of aesthetic concerns as function is only affected in more severe cases.

Deciduous dentition

In severe hypodontia or anodontia early treatment may involve the placement of dentures to help improve aesthetics and function. These can be placed at a very young age but are especially important psychologically just before the start of the school years.

Mixed dentition

Dental development should be closely monitored and a high index of suspicion should be maintained for maxillary canine impaction when the lateral incisors are mis-shapen or absent (see Chapter 32). The psychological impact of hypodontia may not be apparent until eruption of the permanent incisors when the child may notice spacing and may be teased at school. If this is significant, it may be appropriate to build up microdont teeth with composite resin to help close space or provide dentures to replace missing anterior teeth. Simple orthodontic treatment can also be considered (e.g. diastema closure), but this does then commit the patient to retention for a number of years until definitive orthodontics is commenced.

Permanent dentition

Once in the permanent dentition, patients will require a **joint orthodontic–prosthodontic assessment**. Generally speaking, cases with severe hypodontia require more prosthodontic than orthodontic input whilst milder cases can sometimes be treated with the use of orthodontics alone.

Fixed appliance treatment is often undertaken to correct any superimposed malocclusion, **close** or **open** missing tooth spaces and to make **roots parallel** for later implant treatment (Figure 33.1B). A **trial diagnostic (Kesling) set-up**, using duplicate study models, can be used to predict the final aesthetic and occlusal outcome for different treatment options. In some cases, it maybe feasible to keep retained deciduous teeth, especially the second deciduous molars, if these have a good long-term prognosis. Factors influencing the long-term prognosis of retained deciduous teeth include caries, toothwear, root resorption and infraocclusion. An advantage of keeping these teeth include their ability to maintain alveolar bone height.

A prosthodontic opinion should be obtained *before* orthodontic debond to ensure that teeth have been positioned ideally for restorative treatment. Long-cone periapical radiographs should be obtained at potential sites of implant placement to ensure that roots have been separated adequately. Following orthodontics, **retention** is important for space maintenance.

In patients with severe hypodontia, removable **dentures** or overdentures may be the most effective treatment option until implant retained prostheses can be offered following cessation of facial growth.

34 Supernumerary teeth

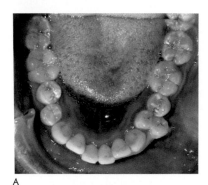

A

Table 34.1 A comparison of the different types of supernumerary teeth.

	Conical	Tuberculate	Supplemental	Odontomes
Occurrence	75%	12%	7%	6%
Shape	Conical shape Complete roots	Barrel shaped Incomplete roots	Resemble normal teeth	Irregular mass or denticles
Site	Anterior maxilla; usually solitary	Anterior maxilla; usually paired	Commonly the upper lateral incisors lower premolars	Anterior maxilla; posterior mandible
Features	Commonly unerupted; maybe inverted; or may erupt	Impede incisor eruption	May erupt	Remain unerupted; can impede eruption

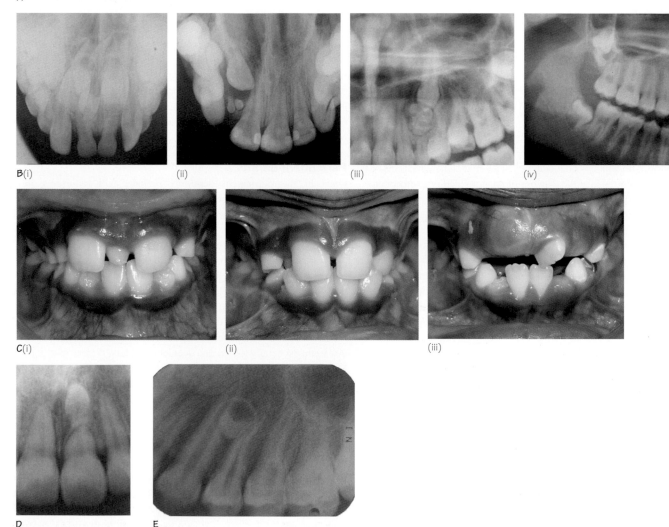

B(i)   (ii)   (iii)   (iv)

C(i)   (ii)   (iii)

D   E

Figure 34.1 (**A**) A supplemental lower left premolar. (**B**) Examples of supernumerary teeth impeding the eruption of premanent teeth. (i) Multiple supernumeraries preventing eruption of the maxillary central incisors, (ii) an odontome in the line of eruption of the upper right permanent lateral incisor, (iii) an odontome impeding the eruption of the upper left permanent canine and (iv) a supernumerary obstructing the eruption of the upper right third molar. (**C**) (i) A mesiodens causing lateral displacement of both central incisors. (ii) Six months after removal there has been spontaneous improvement in incisor position. (iii) An unerupted mesiodens causing rotation of the upper left central incisor. (**D**) An inverted conical supernumerary causing root resorption of the upper left central incisor. (**E**) A late-forming upper premolar.

Supernumerary teeth are defined as teeth in excess of the normal series. Males are twice as commonly affected than females with the following reported prevalences:
- **0.3–0.8%** in the primary dentition;
- **0.1–3.8%** in the permanent dentition.

Supernumerary teeth occur 10 times more frequently in the maxilla than the mandible, with the premaxilla being most commonly affected followed by the mandibular premolar region. A supernumerary tooth in the primary dentition is likely to be followed by a supernumerary in the permanent dentition.

Etiology

Both genetic and environmental factors are probably involved in the development of supernumerary teeth. Developmentally, these teeth are thought to form due to hyperactivity of the dental lamina. Genetic factors may explain why supernumerary teeth can run in families, why males are more commonly affected than females and why supernumeraries can be associated with certain medical conditions.

Classification

Supernumerary teeth can be classified into four groups based on their morphology:
- Conical;
- Tuberculate;
- Supplemental;
- Odontomes.

Table 34.1 compares these four groups. **Conical** supernumeraries are the most common, often occur in the premaxilla and are termed mesiodens when they occur in the midline. Root formation is often complete and sometimes they erupt but can remain unerupted. **Tuberculate** supernumeraries are barrel shaped, consist of multiple tubercles, are often paired and occur in the premaxilla. They form palatal to the central incisors, have incomplete root formation, and often impede the eruption of the central incisors. **Supplemental** supernumeraries resemble teeth of the normal series and most commonly occur in the maxillary lateral incisor region followed by the mandibular premolar region (Figure 34.1A). **Odontomes** maybe **complex** or **compound**. Complex odontomes consist of irregular masses of dental tissue whilst compound odontomes consist of well-organised tooth-like structures.

Clinical features

Supernumerary teeth may remain unnoticed or present as incidental radiographic findings. Sometimes a complication due to their presence may be a presenting feature. Complications include:
- Failure of eruption (Figure 34.1B) – any tooth can be affected where a supernumerary tooth lies in the path of eruption. This is the most common cause of failure of eruption of maxillary central incisors.
- Formation of a midline diastema – a mesiodens may prevent approximation of the central incisor roots with resultant diastema formation.
- Crowding – erupted supernumerary teeth may take up arch space and evidence suggests that there is a generalised increase in tooth size in patients with supernumerary teeth.
- Displacement or rotation of adjacent teeth (Figure 34.1C).
- Root resorption of neighbouring teeth (Figure 34.1D).
- Cystic change within the follicle of the supernumerary tooth and/or migration into adjacent structures.
- Prevention of tooth movement – the presence of a supernumerary tooth may prevent orthodontic movement of adjacent teeth, be a rare cause of incomplete space closure or damage the roots of colliding teeth.

Associated medical conditions

A number of medical conditions may be associated with the presence of supernumerary teeth:
- **Cleft palate ± lip** – supernumerary teeth may form at the site of the cleft.
- **Cleidocranial dysplasia** – this is a rare autosomal dominantly inherited disorder with clinical features that include aplasia or agenesis of the clavicles, Class III malocclusion and the presence of multiple supernumeraries (Figure 13.1Eiii). The supernumeraries may contribute to failure of eruption of permanent teeth.
- **Gardner's syndrome** – this is a rare autosomal dominantly inherited disorder with features that include premalignant polyposis of the large intestine, multiple osteomas of the facial bones, skin tumours and multiple supernumerary teeth.

Management

The first stage of management is the **localisation** and identification of **complications** associated with supernumeraries. Teeth can be localised using the vertical or horizontal parallax technique (Figure 32.1B). A periapical radiograph taken using the paralleling technique gives the most detailed assessment compared with other radiographic views.

If teeth are causing no complications and are not likely to interfere with orthodontic tooth movement they can be **monitored** with yearly radiographic review. The patient should be warned of complications such as cystic change and migration with damage to nearby roots. If the patient does not wish to risk such complications, it is acceptable to remove supernumerary teeth. If they are associated with the roots of permanent teeth it is often sensible to await full root development before surgical extraction to prevent damage to Hertwig's epithelial root sheath. Root development of the maxillary incisors should be complete by the age of 10 years.

If supernumerary teeth are associated with **complications**, it is usual to **extract** such teeth which usually involves a surgical procedure. Early extraction of supernumeraries causing incisor impaction may have the benefit of minimising loss of eruptive potential, space loss and centre-line displacement. One disadvantage of early removal is the risk of root damage to adjacent teeth. After removal, an impacted incisor may take an average of 20 months to erupt (range 7–36 months) and in 50% of cases the tooth may not erupt. It is therefore recommended that unerupted incisors are also exposed and bonded at the time of supernumerary tooth removal and that a **space maintainer** is fitted whilst awaiting spontaneous eruption.

If supernumerary teeth are likely to interfere with **orthodontic tooth movement**, they should be removed prior to the commencement of treatment.

If a **supplemental tooth** is present and erupted, it may be difficult to determine which is the supplemental and which is the tooth of the normal dental series. In these circumstances, assuming both teeth are healthy, it is logical to extract the tooth most displaced from the line of the arch for the relief of crowding.

Finally, the presence of a supernumerary tooth should alert the clinician to the possibility of the development of **late forming supernumerary teeth** especially in the lower premolar region. It has been reported that up to **20%** of patients with an anterior maxillary supernumerary tooth may later develop supplemental premolars (Figure 34.1E).

Treatment techniques

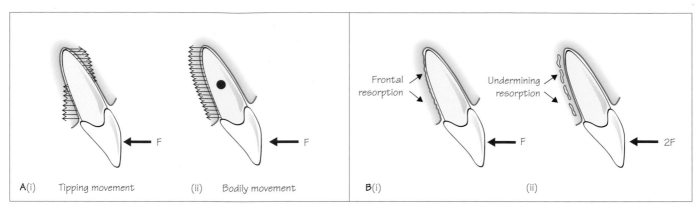

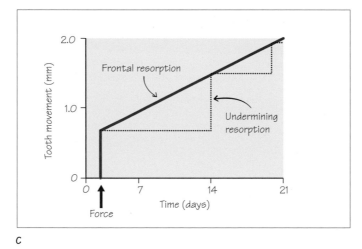

Table 35.1 Optimal force levels for various tooth movements.

Tooth movement	Force level (g)
Tipping	30–60
Bodily movement	60–120
Rotation	30–60
Extrusion	30–60
Intrusion	10–20

Figure 35.1 (A) (i) Tipping movement results from compressive forces on diagonally opposite ends of the periodontal ligament. These are greatest at the alveolar crest and root apex and reduce to zero adjacent to the centre of resistance. Tension is created in other areas of the periodontal ligament. (ii) Bodily movement results from even compressive forces along one side of the periodontal ligament and tension on the opposite side. (B) (i) Frontal resorption occurs when orthodontic forces do not exceed capillary pressure. (ii) Undermining resorption occurs when capillary pressure is exceeded and hyalinisation occurs within the periodontal ligament. (C) Tooth movement occurring during the application of light (frontal resorption) and heavy (undermining resorption) forces. Undermining resorption results in delayed, large tooth movements because a great thickness of alveolar bone must be removed before the bone that lines the alveolar socket is resorbed. If force levels are maintained this process continues to repeat itself.

The application of a continuous force to a tooth results in remodelling of alveolar bone, reorganisation of the periodontal ligament and tooth movement. Orthodontic tooth movement is a complex process that involves the co-ordinated activity of many cell types and numerous chemical mediators. This chapter provides a summary of the mechanism of orthodontic tooth movement.

Effects of force on the periodontal ligament

The application of a continuous force to a tooth surface results in the development of areas of compression and tension within the periodontal ligament (Figure 35.1A). **Tipping** forces produce compressive loads that are greatest at the alveolar crest and root apex on diagonally opposite sides. **Bodily** movement results from even compressive loads along one side of the periodontal ligament.

The magnitude of the force delivered is important in determining the tissue response. Ideally, orthodontic forces should not exceed the **capillary pressure** within the periodontal ligament as this produces ischemia and tissue necrosis. The optimal force for tooth movement also depends on the type of tooth movement planned and the root surface area of the teeth to be moved – teeth with smaller roots require less force for movement than teeth with larger roots. Table 35.1 outlines the **ideal force levels** for various tooth movements. The forces required for bodily movement are double those required for tipping as double the root surface area is compressed on one side during bodily movement. The forces for intrusion are the lightest because all the force is concentrated at the root apex which has a small surface area.

Light orthodontic forces that do not exceed capillary pressure result in **frontal bone resorption** in areas of compression and deposition in areas of tension.

Forces that exceed capillary pressure result in sterile necrosis in the area of the periodontal ligament affected. This process is termed **hyalinisation** because the area appears translucent when viewed under the light microscope. Orthodontic tooth movement is delayed and bone resorption commences from beneath the area of necrosis within a few days. This is termed **undermining resorption** because the cellular response occurs from the narrow spaces on the undersurface of the area of necrosis.

Cellular responses to orthodontic forces

Cellular responses are evident within the periodontal ligament after a few hours from the initiation of an orthodontic force. Altered gene expression may be triggered by changes in the local blood flow and/or the mechanical deformation of cells. Many chemical mediators have been detected within the tissues following force application including prostaglandin E, cytokines and nitric oxide. The role of individual chemical mediators is poorly understood.

Osteoclasts, derived from monocyte-hematopoietic cells, appear on the alveolar bone surface adjacent to the areas of compression within approximately 48 hours of force application. These cells resorb the surface of the alveolar bone, in a process termed **frontal resorption** (Figure 35.1Bi), which marks the commencement of tooth movement. The term *frontal* is used to denote that bone resorption occurs from *in front* of the root.

Osteoblasts are recruited from stem cells within the periodontal ligament and appear in areas of tension and deposit bone matrix approximately 48 hours after force application. As bone resorption occurs more rapidly than deposition, there is slight widening of the periodontal space during tooth movement. The periodontal ligament also undergoes considerable remodelling, with resorption of existing fibres and deposition of new fibres, mediated by **fibrobasts** present within the ligament.

When orthodontic forces exceed capillary pressure, tissue necrosis occurs and undermining resorption is carried out by cell populations derived from the marrow spaces of the alveolar bone (Figure 35.1Bii). Resorption of the necrotic tissue also leads to resorption of root surface cementum adjacent to these areas, by cells termed **cementoclasts**, and may be the mechanism causing orthodontically related **root resorption**. Areas of resorbed cementum may undergo repair if the defects are small. With prolonged heavy forces, root resorption may outstrip deposition and there may be significant root shortening (Figure 12.1C).

It takes approximately 7–14 days for the process of undermining resorption to remove the lamina dura next to the necrotic periodontal ligament which is the point at which tooth movement occurs (Figure 35.1C). It is difficult to avoid undermining resorption even when care is taken during force application. This is because a degree of dental tipping is likely to occur within the socket that will result in the concentration of forces at the root apex and alveolar crest (Figure 35.1Ai). A time period of at least 4–6 weeks is recommended between appliance reactivation appointments to allow adequate time for repair of damaged tissues whilst the active forces from the appliance have declined.

Orthodontically related **pain** may result from the inflammatory response that normally accompanies **tissue necrosis**. **Neurogenic inflammation** may also be an important factor because nerve endings within the periodontal ligament release mediators (e.g. calcitonin gene-related peptide, substance P) that trigger an inflammatory response during force application. A transient **pulpitis** may also accompany force application which may contribute to the pain sensation.

The rate of tooth movement

Ideally, orthodontic forces should be applied for a 24 hours/day in order to produce the most efficient rate of tooth movement. Clinical experience suggests that at least 6 hours/day of force must be delivered to produce minimal movement.

Under ideal conditions, the rate of tooth movement is approximately **1 mm/month**. There is **individual variation** as the rate depends on the efficiency and magnitude of the cellular response and the density of the alveolar bone. The initiation of tooth movement may be slower in **adults** because of the reduced cellularity and vascularity of the periodontal ligament and the greater density of the alveolar bone compared to children. Tooth movement through cancellous bone is more rapid than movement through cortical bone.

Mechanisms linking force application to tooth movement

Two main theories have been proposed to explain the link between orthodontic force application and the cellular responses that lead to tooth movement:

• Pressure–tension theory;
• Bioelectric theory.

The **pressure–tension theory** suggests that areas of pressure and tension generated within the periodontal ligament result in alterations in blood flow, which triggers the release of chemical messengers that further trigger the cellular reactions associated with tooth movement. The **bioelectric theory** links bending of the alveolar bone, during force application, to the generation of electrical currents which trigger the desired cellular events. It is not clear which of these theories is more valid, and it is possible that both mechanisms may contribute to orthodontic tooth movement.

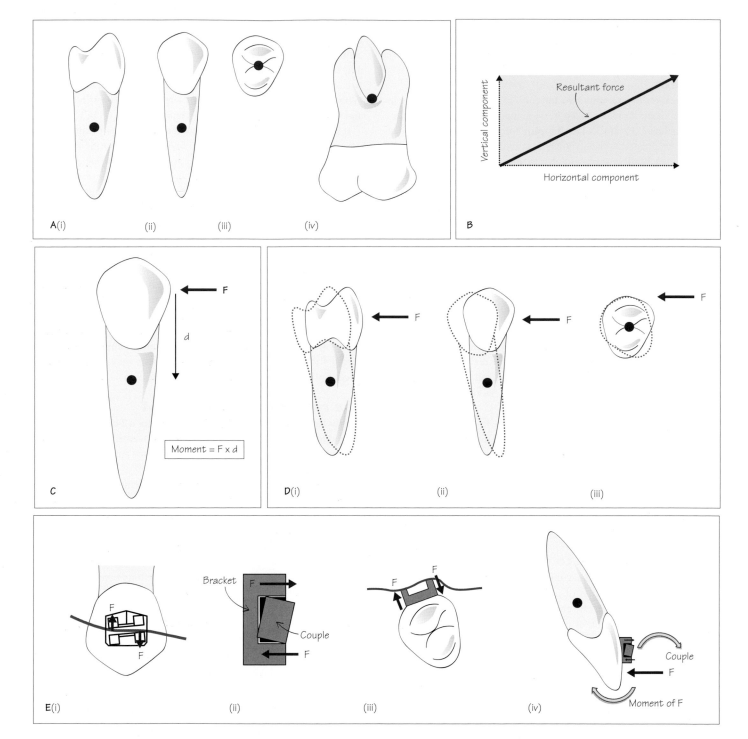

Figure 36.1 (**A**) The centre of resistance (red circle) of a single-rooted tooth shown in the (i) buccolingual, (ii) mesiodistal and (iii) occlusal plane. (iv) The centre of resistance of a molar is located in the furcation region. (**B**) The resultant force can be broken down into its various components. Here the resultant force has both a horizontal and vertical component that will influence the direction of tooth movement. (**C**) The size of a moment is equal to the magnitude of the force (F) multiplied by the distance from the tooth's centre of resistance (d) from which it acts . (**D**) Forces applied at a distance from the centre of resistance result in rotation of the tooth. This should be considered in all planes of space: (i) buccolingual, (ii) mesiodistal and (iii) occlusal. (**E**) An archwire in a bracket slot can be used to apply a couple in the: (i) mesiodistal, (ii) buccopalatal, and (iii) occlusal planes. (iv) The couple created between the bracket slot and archwire can be used to control the tipping caused by the moment of the force (F). In this way, bodily tooth movement can be achieved.

Biomechanics is the science concerned with the effects of forces acting on the human body. A basic understanding of the biomechanics of tooth movement will help the reader to understand the effects an applied force will have on the direction of tooth movement.

Centre of resistance

Single teeth, groups of teeth and the facial bones have a centre of resistance. This is the point in a body at which resistance to movement is concentrated. If a force is applied directly to the centre of resistance of an object, bodily movement will occur. For a restrained object, such as a tooth, the centre of resistance does not coincide with the centre of mass and is determined by the shape of the tooth and properties of the alveolar bone and periodontal ligament.

The centre of resistance should be visualised in all planes of space (Figure 36.1A). For a single rooted tooth, with normal periodontal attachment, the centre of resistance is approximately halfway down the root surface. For multi-rooted teeth the equivalent point is in the area of the root furcation. Alveolar bone loss results in apical movement of the centre of resistance.

The centre of resistance of the maxilla is thought to lie in the area of the premolar roots. It is an important point to appreciate when applying headgear forces for maxillary restraint.

Forces, moments and couples

Orthodontic tooth movement is dependent on the application of forces. A **force** is a vector that can be described by its magnitude and direction and can be broken down into its individual components (Figure 36.1B). This can help determine the effects a force will have on the direction of tooth movement.

The **moment** of a force is the component of the force that tends to cause rotation. Mathematically, the size of a moment of a force is equal to the magnitude of the applied force multiplied by the perpendicular distance between the point of application and the centre of resistance (Figure 36.1C). This is of relevance to orthodontics because a force cannot be applied directly to a tooth's centre of resistance, which lies along the root, and must be applied to the crown. This will produce a moment which will cause the tooth to rotate (Figure 36.1D).

A **couple** is produced when two equal and opposite forces act to cause rotation. The size of a couple is equal to the magnitude of the forces applied multiplied by the distance between them. Couples are commonly generated during fixed appliance treatment between an archwire and bracket slot (Figure 36.1Ei–iii). They can be used to alter the inclination of teeth or to act in the opposite direction to the moment of an applied force to produce bodily tooth movement (Figure 36.1Eiv). The term **torque** is often used in orthodontics to describe a moment or couple.

Types of tooth movement

The basic types of tooth movement are tipping, bodily movement and rotation.

Tipping occurs when the crown of a tooth moves more than its root in a given direction. This form of movement is common during orthodontic treatment as the moment created by the applied force will tend to cause tipping. It is important to remember that when a tooth tips, the crown and root move in opposite directions.

Bodily movement occurs when the crown and root of a tooth move an equal distance in the same direction. This type of tooth movement can only be produced with fixed appliances where a couple can be created between an archwire and the wall of a bracket slot to control tipping that accompanies the application on an orthodontic force to the crown of a tooth.

When a mesial or distal force is applied to the labial surface of a tooth, the moment of the force will cause **rotation**. This is commonly encountered during fixed appliance treatment. It is good practice to tie teeth firmly to the archwire to prevent unwanted rotation, when such forces are applied.

Table 37.1 The magnitude and duration of headgear forces required for anchorage reinforcement, distalisation of maxillary molars and maxillary restraint.

	Anchorage	Distal movement	Maxillary restraint
Force	250–300 g	400–500 g	500+ g
Duration	10–12h	12+h	12+h

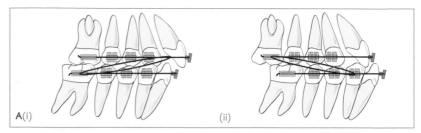

A(i)   (ii)

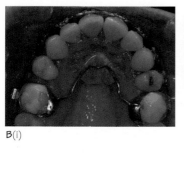

B(i)

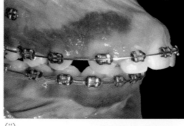

(ii)

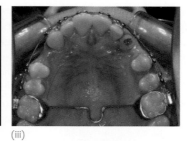

(iii)

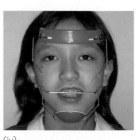

(iv)

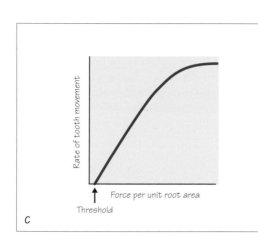

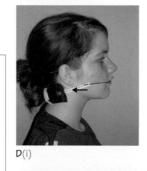

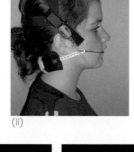

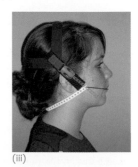

D(i)   (ii)   (iii)

C

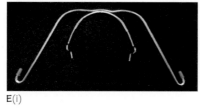

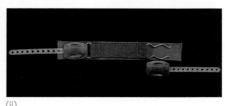

E(i)   (ii)

Figure 37.1 (**A**) Intermaxillary traction. (i) Class II elastics run from the lower molars to the upper incisors. They aid upper incisor retraction and mesial lower molar movement whilst maintaining the upper molar and lower incisor position. There is also an extrusive force placed onto the lower molars and upper incisors. (ii) Class III elastics run from the upper molars to the lower incisors and encourage lower incisor retraction and mesial movement of the upper molars whilst maintaining the position of the upper incisors and lower molars. (**B**) Anchorage appliances. Clinical examples (i) Nance palatal arch, (ii) mini-screw implants (iii) transpalatal arch and (iv) protraction headgear. (**C**) The relationship between the force per unit area of root surface and the rate of orthodontic tooth movement (differential force theory). A threshold force exists below which no tooth movement occurs. (**D**) Examples of headgear (i) low (cervical) pull with a neck strap, (ii) straight pull using a head and neck strap and (iii) high pull using a head strap. The red arrow shows the Masel safety strap. (**E**) Components of headgear: (i) the Kloehn bow, (ii) snap-away elastic modules. The neck strap, head strap and Masel safety strap (arrow) are shown in Figure (Di).

Anchorage maybe defined as resistance to the unwanted three dimensional forces generated in reaction to the active components of an appliance. The reactive forces are equal and opposite to the active forces according to Newton's third law of motion (every action produces an equal and opposite reaction). Poor anchorage management can result in a non-ideal occlusion, over-retraction or under-retraction of the incisors, and poor facial aesthetics.

Anchorage requirements should be assessed by **space analysis** during treatment planning (Chapter 18). If 75–100% of extraction space is required for the correction of malocclusion, anchorage requirements can be considered to be high.

Classification of anchorage devices

Anchorage devices can be classified according to the tissue(s) providing resistance to unwanted tooth movement.

Intra-orally the teeth, skeletal structures and soft tissues can provide anchorage. When the **teeth** are used, the anchor unit should incorporate as many teeth as possible, so that the force threshold needed to initiate tooth movement is not exceeded. Teeth from the opposing dental arch can also be used to provide inter-arch anchorage with Class II or III intermaxillary elastics (Figure 37.1A). The **bone** covering the palate can be a useful source of anchorage because of its large surface area. Removable appliances and the Nance palatal arch (Figure 37.1Bi) commonly use the palate as a source of anchorage. More recently, **skeletal** anchorage has become increasingly popular with the introduction of implants and mini-screws (Figure 37.1Bii). These devices provide **maximum anchorage**, unlike previously mentioned methods, which means that space loss is minimal. These methods can be used in high anchorage cases. The transpalatal arch (Figure 37.1Biii), which connects the maxillary first permanent molars, uses the cortical bone for anchorage. This appliance maintains the inter-molar width so that as the molars migrate anteriorly with anchorage loss, their roots contact the buccal cortical plate (as the maxilla gets narrower anteriorly) which provides greater resistance to tooth movement (cortical anchorage). In practice, the transpalatal arch provides minimal anteroposterior anchorage.

Extra-oral appliances use the cranium or facial skeleton to resist the reactive forces. **Retraction headgear** (see later) can be used in highly anchorage demanding cases and to distalise the maxillary molars. **Protraction headgear** (Figure 37.1Biv) can be used for space closure by mesial maxillary molar movement to avoid maxillary incisor retraction (Class III malocclusion). Successful anchorage management with extra-oral devices relies on high levels of patient compliance.

Factors determining anchorage value

Initially a linear relationship exists between the **force per unit area generated on the root surface** by the active components of an appliance and the rate of tooth movement (Figure 37.1C). A threshold force exists below which no tooth movement will occur (differential force theory). Therefore, one principle of anchorage management is to incorporate as many teeth into an **anchorage unit** as possible, to distribute the reactive forces over as large a root surface area and to keep the **active forces as low as possible**. Consideration can also be given to moving teeth in stages (e.g. canine retraction) to minimise the active forces required. Following these principles will help to reduce space loss in cases where anchorage control is critical.

The **type of tooth movement** influences the anchorage required. Bodily movement requires more active force than tipping movement (Table 35.1) and is therefore more anchorage demanding. The anchorage value of teeth can be increased by minimising tipping during fixed appliance treatment.

The **extraction pattern** can influence anchorage balance and minimise unwanted tooth movement during fixed appliance treatment. For example, a favourable extraction pattern in some (not all) Class II cases is the loss of upper first premolars and lower second premolars. This helps to increase the number of teeth in the posterior maxillary anchorage unit which maximises incisor retraction. In the lower arch, the number of anchor teeth in the lower anterior mandibular segment is increased which helps to minimise incisor retraction and maximise mesial molar movement. The use of Class II intermaxillary traction facilitates upper incisor retraction and mesial movement of the lower molars whilst maintaining the position of the lower incisors. In Class III cases, upper second and lower first premolar extractions are preferred as the anchorage balance favours minimal upper incisor and maximal lower incisor retraction. The use of Class III intermaxillary traction favours these movements.

Bone quality can influence the anchorage value of teeth. Dense mandibular bone offers more resistance to tooth movement than maxillary bone. As a result, space closure in the mandibular arch during fixed appliance treatment often lags behind that in the maxillary arch. Cancellous bone offers less resistance to tooth movement than denser cortical bone. Anchorage loss can be reduced by moving the roots of anchor teeth closer to the cortical plate (cortical anchorage). However, this may predispose to greater root resorption.

The **vertical facial dimension** can influence the rate of tooth movement. Space or anchorage loss occurs more rapidly in patients with an increased face height. This may be due to a number of factors including a more mesial path of molar eruption in those with an increased MMPA (the lower molars erupt at 90° to the mandibular plane) and less occlusal interlocking.

Good buccal **interdigitation and occlusal interferences** can reduce the rate of tooth movement. However, in anchor teeth good interdigitation may be favourable.

Facial growth and anchorage management

Growth during orthodontic treatment can positively or negatively influence anchorage management. For example, favourable forwards mandibular growth in Class II malocclusion can help to reduce the overjet and anchorage requirements for upper incisor retraction. However, unfavourable mandibular growth (clockwise (backward) rotation) can increase the overjet which raises anchorage requirements in the maxilla. Downwards and backwards rotation of the mandible in Class III malocclusion can be favourable by helping overjet correction and reducing anchorage requirements for lower incisor retraction. However, unfavourable forwards mandibular growth during treatment can have the reverse effect.

Headgear

Retraction headgear can provide maximum anchorage assuming good patient compliance. It can be used to:
- prevent mesial movement of the maxillary molars (**extra-oral anchorage**);
- move the maxillary molars distally with or without vertical movement (**extra-oral traction**);
- restrain maxillary growth (growth modification).

The effect produced depends on the **magnitude, duration** and **direction** of the headgear force (Table 37.1). Higher forces and more daily wear, increase the amount of tooth movement and maxillary restraint. The direction of headgear force can be:
- **low (cervical) pull** in relationship to the occlusal plane;
- **straight pull** and parallel to the occlusal plane;
- **high pull** in relationship to the occlusal plane.

Low (cervical) pull headgear (Figure 37.1Di) places both extrusive and distalising forces onto the first molars and is useful in those with a reduced facial height and deep overbite. Straight-pull headgear (Figure 37.1Dii) places distalising forces only and can be used in patients with a normal face height. High-pull headgear (Figure 37.1Diii) places both intrusive and distalising forces onto the first molars and can be used in patient with an increased vertical dimension.

The components of headgear are shown in Figures 37.1D and 37.1E. Forces are commonly applied with the Kloehn bow (Figure 37.1Ei) attached to an upper removable appliance or bands placed onto the maxillary first permanent molars. The **safety** components include the Masel safety strap (Figure 37.1Di), snap-away force delivery modules (Figure 37.1Eii), recurved and locking Kloehn bows. At least two of these safety mechanisms should be used together to reduce the risk of **ocular injury** and blindness. Such injuries can occur if the Kloehn bow is dislodged from the mouth and catapults back into the face.

Table 38.1
Commonly used active components of removable appliances and their uses.

Active components	Fabrication (ss, stainless steel wire)	Use
Labial movement		
Double cantilever spring (Z-spring)	0.5–0.6 mm diameter ss	Proclination of 1 or 2 incisors (good range) (Activate by pulling away from baseplate at 45°)
T-spring	0.5–0.6 mm diameter ss	Proclination of an incisor/premolar/molar (poor range) (Activate by pulling away from baseplate at 45°)
Recurved spring	0.8 mm diameter ss	Proclination of all four incisors
Cross-over wires	0.7–0.8 mm diameter ss	Proclination of all four incisors
Screws	–	Proclination of multiple incisors where retention poor
Palatal movement		
Roberts' retractor	0.5 mm diameter ss (sleeved)	Retraction of prolined and spaced maxillary incisors
Buccal canine retractor	0.5 mm (sleeved) or 0.7 mm diameter ss (unsleeved)	Palatal and distal movement of mesially angulated canines
Elastics	Different diameters available	Force dependent on the root surface area of teeth to be moved
Distal movement		
Palatal finger spring	0.5–0.7 mm diameter ss (guarded)	Distal movement of canines, premolars and molars
Headgear	–	Distal movement of molars, J-hook headgear for incisor retraction
Expansion		
Screw	–	Correction of buccal crossbites
Coffin spring	1.25 mm diameter ss	Buccal crossbite correction
Rotation		
Whip spring	0.5 mm diameter ss	Correction of mild rotations
Extrusion and Intrusion		
Elastics	Different diameters available	Force dependent on the root surface area of teeth to be moved

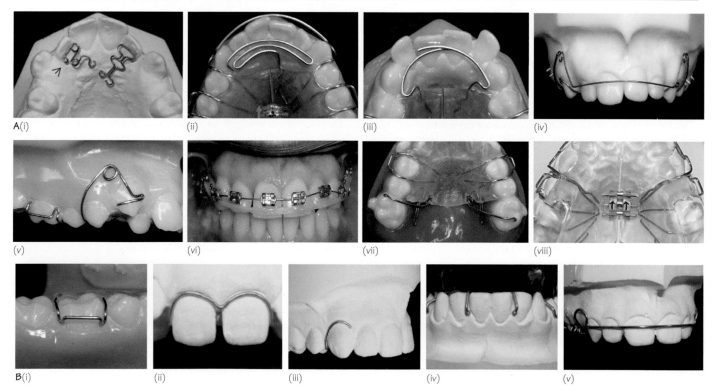

Figure 38.1 (**A**) Examples of active removable appliance components: (i) Z-spring (arrow) and T-spring, (ii) recurved spring, (iii) cross-over wires, (iv) Roberts retractor, (v) buccal canine retractor, (vi) elastics, (vii) palatal finger spring for distal molar movement and (viii) midline expansion screw. (**B**) Examples of retentive removable appliance components: (i) Adams clasp, (ii) Southend clasp, (iii) C(ircumferential)-clasp, (iv) ball ended clasps and (v) labial bow.

A removable appliance is an appliance that can be removed by the patient for the maintenance of oral hygiene. Appliances maybe active, when designed to move teeth, or passive, when used as retainers (see Chapter 41) or space maintainers (see Chapter 28). Functional appliances may be removable or fixed and are described in Chapter 39.

The use of removable appliances has declined in recent times because of the higher-quality results obtained with fixed appliances. The relative advantages and disadvantages of fixed and removable appliances are summarised in Table 39.1. The role of upper removable appliances for tooth movement in modern orthodontics includes:
• interceptive treatment during the mixed dentition (e.g. crossbite correction);
• facilitation of distal movement of the molars using headgear (e.g. the nudger and *en masse* appliance);
• as an adjunct to fixed appliance treatment (e.g. anterior bite planes for overbite reduction);
• maxillary restraint (e.g. maxillary intrusion splint);
• assess motivation and compliance before more complex treatment.

Lower removable appliances are rarely used for tooth movement as they are poorly tolerated due to lack of retention. This is often due to poor undercuts on the molars and tongue activity.

Components of removable appliances

The component of a removable appliance can be recalled by remembering the acronym ARAB:
• **A**ctive components;
• **R**etentive components;
• **A**nchorage;
• **B**aseplate.

Active components

The active components generate the forces that result in tooth movement and may be springs, screws or elastics (Table 38.1, Figure 38.1A). **Springs** (Figure 38.1A) are the most commonly used active component and are constructed from hard polished stainless steel. The force (F) delivered by a spring can be calculated using the following formula: $F \propto dr^4/l^3$, where d = deflection; r = radius; l = length.

Small changes in diameter and length have a large effect on the force delivered: doubling the radius increases the force 16-fold and doubling the length reduces the force eight-fold. Coils can be placed into springs to increase their length which reduces the force delivered and increases the range. Ideally, a spring should deliver a light force over a long range. As a general rule a spring should be activated by half a tooth width and should be reactivated every 6–8 weeks.

Screws (Figure 38.1Aviii) are an alternative method of delivering active forces. In contrast with springs, which are generally used to move single units, screws can be used to move groups of teeth. An advantage of a screw is that the teeth to be moved can be clasped if retention is a problem. Disadvantages include very high forces on activation that dissipate rapidly. Typically, a quarter turn will produce 0.25 mm of expansion and reactivation should occur weekly.

Orthodontic **elastics** (Figure 38.1Avi) are occasionally used to deliver active forces. Latex-free varieties should be used for patients allergic to this material. Elastics are supplied in many different diameters and are capable of delivering different levels of forces (e.g. 2 oz, 3.5 oz). Generally, stretching the elastic to three times its diameter will deliver the force levels shown on the packet. Ideally, these should be checked using a strain gauge (e.g. Correx gauge) to confirm the correct level. The prescribed force will depend on the root surface area of the teeth to be moved. Advantages of elastics include their relatively good aesthetics and their ability to apply intrusive, extrusive as well as distalising force. Disadvantages include the force levels diminish rapidly intra-orally, wear is dependent on good compliance and they often snap during use.

Retentive components

Retention is the resistance to displacement away from the tissues. It is essential that appliances are retentive to enable the active components to work efficiently and for patient comfort. A number of components are available to provide retention.

Adams clasps (Figure 38.1Bi) can be placed onto any tooth but are usually used on first permanent molars, the first premolars or the first deciduous molar teeth. The arrow-head engages the mesiobuccal and distobuccal undercuts. Clasps on primary teeth can be constructed from 0.6 mm diameter stainless steel wire, single clasps on permanent teeth from 0.7 mm diameter stainless steel wire and double clasps or single clasps used to accept headgear from 0.8 mm diameter stainless steel wire.

Anterior retention can be gained by using the **Southend clasp** (0.7 mm diameter stainless steel wire, Figure 38.1Bii) which engages the undercut beneath the contact point between the maxillary central incisors. A disadvantage of this clasp is its visibility. The **C(ircumferential)-clasp** (0.6–0.8 mm diameter stainless steel wire, Figure 38.1Biii) can be used to engage the interproximal gingival undercut of the canines or molars. An advantage of this clasp is the possibility of avoiding occlusal interference on one side. The **ball-ended clasp** (0.7–0.8 mm diameter stainless steel wire, Figure 38.1Biv) crosses the occlusal/incisal surface between two adjacent teeth and engages the mesiobuccal and distobuccal undercuts. They are commonly used between the lower incisors for anterior retention or the upper premolars when a removable appliance is used in conjunction with a fixed appliance. A **labial bow** (0.7 mm diameter stainless steel wire, Figure 37.1Bv) can be used to help retain an upper removable appliance especially if the incisors are proclined. It can also be used to guide the movement of teeth when used with other active components. A major disadvantage is its high visibility.

Anchorage

The principles of anchorage are discussed in Chapter 37. An advantage of removable appliances are their good anchorage control. This is largely because unwanted reactive forces are dissipated over the palatal tissues, many teeth can be incorporated into the anchorage unit and active forces can be kept light. As well as anteroposterior anchorage, removable appliances provide good vertical and reciprocal transverse anchorage. Anchorage can also be supplemented with headgear.

Baseplate

The baseplate is usually constructed from cold-cured polymethylmethacrylate but can be made from heat-cured material when high strength is required (e.g. high occlusal forces). It has a number of functions including housing and protecting the active and retentive components and transmitting the reactive forces to the palate and anchor teeth. Additional functions include the formation of **anterior and posterior bite planes**. Flat anterior bite planes are used for overbite reduction, by molar extrusion and minimal lower incisor intrusion, in growing patients. They can also be used for the elimination of occlusal interferences that prevent tooth movement during fixed appliance treatment. Posterior bite planes are used to disocclude the anterior teeth for crossbite correction. They should be just thick enough to provide the required separation to remain relatively comfortable.

Mechanism of action

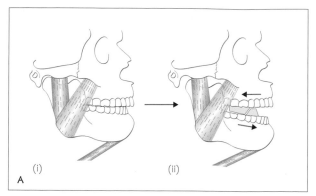

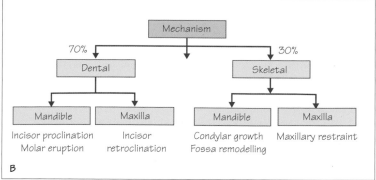

B

The twin block appliance

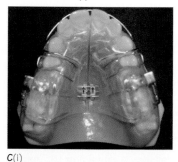

C(i)

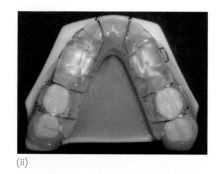

(ii)

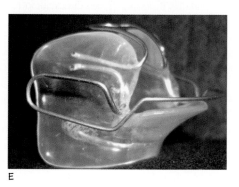

(iii)

The functional regulator II and bionator appliances

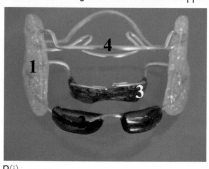

D(i)

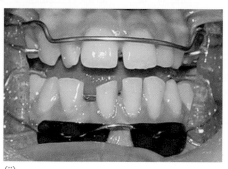

(ii)

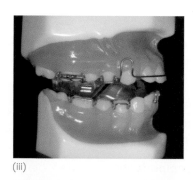

E

Figure 39.1 (**A**) Vertical and anterior posturing of the mandible results in muscular and soft tissue stretching. This produces forces which act on the dentition, through the appliance, to produce tooth movement. (**B**) The mechanism of action of functional appliances. (**C**) The twin block appliance. The (i) upper component, (ii) lower component and (iii) side view. The blocks interdigitate at 45–70° to posture the mandible forwards (note the edge-edge incisor relationship). (**D**) The funtional regulator II appliance: (i) the various components: 1 = buccal shield, 2 = labial pad, 3 = lingual pad and 4 = labial bow. (ii) The functional regulartor II in situ. (**E**) The bionator appliance.

A functional appliance can be defined as an appliance that alters the posture of the mandible, causing stretching of the facial soft tissues, to produce a combination of dental and skeletal changes. Functional appliances are most commonly used in the management of Class II malocclusion, however, they are occasionally used in Class III malocclusion. This chapter will focus on the use of functional appliances for the treatment of Class II malocclusion.

These appliances may be classified according to whether they are **tooth-borne or mucosa-borne** (e.g. the functional regulator II (FRII)). Tooth-borne appliances maybe classified as passive (e.g. bionator), if they carry no active components, or active (e.g. twin block) if they carry active components such as expansion screws and/or springs.

Patient selection

The following criteria should be fulfilled to prescribe a functional appliance:
• A **significant Class II** skeletal discrepancy with mandibular retrognathia.
• A **growing patient**. Ideally, treatment should be carried out during the pubertal growth spurt (males 14 ± 2 years; females 10 ± 2 years) for maximum response. The magnitude of the skeletal response declines following this.
• A **compliant patient**. Functional appliances can be difficult to tolerate and patients must attend for regular appointments.

Mode of action

Functional appliances work by posturing the mandible forwards, which causes soft tissue stretching. This generates Class II intermaxillary traction forces (Figure 39.1A). The resultant correction in overjet is produced by combination of **tooth movement (70%)** and **skeletal change (30%)** (Figure 39.1B). The effects of functional appliances are:
• **Dentoalveolar changes** – these include retroclination of the maxillary incisors and proclination of the mandibular incisors due to the Class II traction forces developed between the arches, and because the upper incisors come under the control of the lower lip with anterior mandibular posturing.
• **Increased mandibular length** – due to downward and forward translation of the condyle which may encourage backward compensatory growth. In the short term, mandibular length may increase by 2–4 mm although there is great **individual variation**. There is evidence from long-term studies that the early growth benefit may be lost with time.
• **An increase in lower anterior face height (LAFH)** – due to a combination of molar eruption and downwards mandibular growth. This is useful where there is a deep overbite (OB)/short LAFH and detrimental in those with a reduced OB/ increased LAFH.
• **Forward remodeling of the glenoid fossa** – this occurs secondary to anterior condylar repositioning.
• **Restraint of maxillary growth** – due to the Class II traction forces acting on the maxilla. Incorporation of **headgear** into functional appliance treatment increases this effect.

Types of functional appliances

One common feature between all the appliances described below is that they are constructed from a bite registration taken with the mandible postured forwards.

The twin block appliance

The twin block appliance (Figure 39.1C) is suitable for Class II cases with a reduced or normal vertical dimension. High-pull headgear should be used in those with an increased face height to limit vertical maxillary growth. It is a **two-piece appliance** that is intended to be worn full-time. An advantage of the two-piece design is that it allows lateral mandibular excursions during wear that may increase comfort and improve compliance. The **mandibular appliance** (Figure 39.1Cii) consists of an acrylic baseplate with Adams clasps placed onto the first permanent molars and first premolars. The bite blocks cover the occlusal surface of the premolars. The **maxillary appliance** (Figure 39.1Ci) consists of an acrylic baseplate, with a mid-line expansion screw, incorporating Adams clasps in a similar manner to the mandibular appliance. The bite blocks cover the occlusal surface of the premolars and molars. Some clinicians incorporate a labial bow to aid retraction of the maxillary incisors and appliance retention. On insertion of both appliances, the bite blocks, which interdigitate at 45–70°, force the mandible to posture anteriorly (Figure 39.1Ciii).

The functional regulator II appliance

Rolf Frankel described a number of functional regulator appliances of which the functional regulator II is the most popular. Frankel believed that the capacity to regulate facial growth resided in the soft tissues. The appliance aims to remove the restrictive soft tissue forces which limit normal maxillary and mandibular development. The appliance is mainly used in Class II cases with a **lip trap** or in the **mixed dentition** as the appliance is mucosa-borne and retention is not affected by shedding deciduous teeth. The role of the **buccal shields** (Figure 39.1D) is to limit cheek pressure on the maxillary buccal segments and allow expansion under unopposed tongue pressure. The buccal shields are vertically overextended into the buccal sulcus in an attempt to cause **periosteal stretch**, which is thought to encourage lateral maxillary bone deposition. The **labial pad** removes restrictive forces from hyperactive mentalis activity. The **lingual pad** contacts the lingual mucosa creating an avoidance reflex which results in anterior mandibular posturing.

The bionator

The original bionator appliance has undergone numerous modifications but essentially consists of a lingual horseshoe of acrylic with molar facets to posture the mandible forwards and guide molar eruption (Figure 39.1E). A labial bow extends posteriorly to act as a buccal shield. There are a number of designs depending on whether the aim is to open, close or maintain the overbite by encouraging or inhibiting molar and/or incisor eruption.

The Herbst appliance

The Herbst appliance is a **fixed functional appliance** which has the advantage of producing rapid occlusal changes as it cannot be removed by the patient. It consists of a metal framework cemented to the upper and lower arches and connected bilaterally by a piston-and-tube telescopic device that forces the mandible forwards.

Table 40.1 The relative advantages and disadvantages of fixed and removable appliances.

Fixed appliances	Removable appliances
Precise three dimensional control of tooth movement	Less precise control of tooth movement
Bodily tooth movement	Tipping movement
Complex malocclusions	Simple malocclusions
High anchorage requirements	Smaller anchorage requirements
Controlled space closure possible	Controlled space closure difficult
Multiple tooth movements	Fewer tooth movements
Can be used in the upper and lower arches	Retention poor in the lower arch
Simple to correct rotations	More difficult to correct rotations
Oral hygiene can be problematic	Removable for oral hygiene
Not dependent on compliance for wear	Dependent on compliance for wear
Long chairside time	Short chairside time
Require extensive training to manage	Require less training to manage

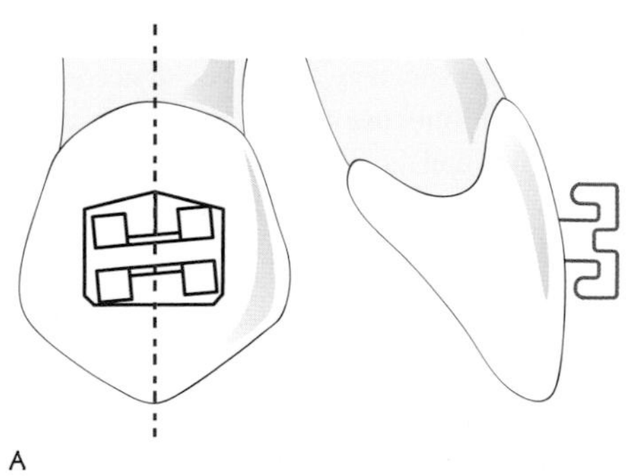

Figure 40.1 (**A**) The mesiodistal tip and inclination of the bracket slot contributes to determining the final tooth position. The bracket should be positioned so that it is parallel to the long axis, and in the midpoint of the crown in order to express the correct built-in value. (**B**) Fixed orthodontic appliances: (i) brackets are placed on the tooth surface. (ii) An archwire is inserted into the bracket slot and (iii) ligated with an elastomeric module. (**C**) Archwires are made from a variety of materials, come in different sizes and can have a round or rectangular cross-section. The wire is formed into a particular archform and will place active forces onto the teeth to move them into this archform. (**D**) Space opening mechanics to create space for the in-standing maxillary lateral incisors. (i) Nickel titanium coil spring used to open the lateral incisor spaces by distal movement of the canines; (ii) once adequate space has been created, a flexible archwire is used to align the teeth; (iii) at the end of alignment.

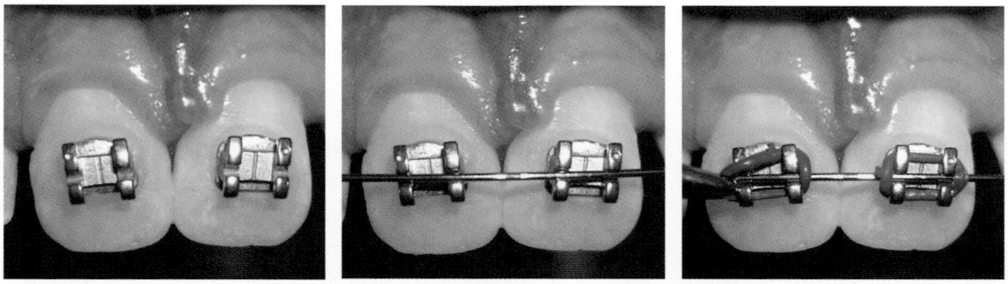

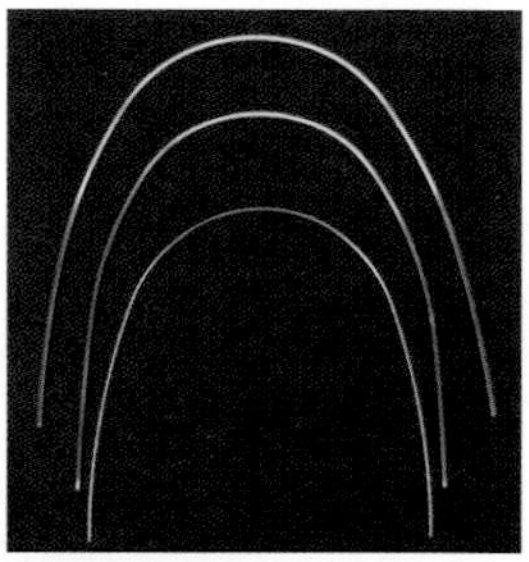

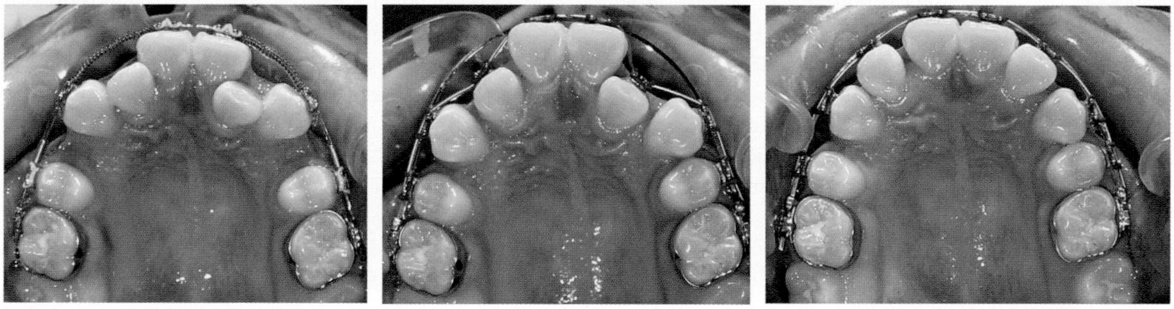

The majority of orthodontic treatment is undertaken with the use of fixed appliances. These have a number of advantages as compared to removable appliance techniques (Table 40.1). There are many fixed appliance systems with the most commonly used being the **'pre-adjusted' edgewise appliance**. This appliance was developed from the standard edgewise appliance that was originally introduced by Edward Angle. The pre-adjusted Edgewise appliance benefits by each tooth having its own individual bracket, with the slot at a specific angle and a base of varying thickness, which positions the tooth at its correct tip/inclination/rotation once a full size archwire has been allowed to fully express itself (Figure 40.1A). This circumvents the requirement for complex archwire bending, which was common practice with the standard Edgewise technique.

The successful use of fixed appliances requires extensive training which is beyond the scope of undergraduate training programmes. General practitioners should, however, have a basic understanding of what these appliances can achieve and the commonly encountered problems.

Components of a fixed appliance

Brackets (Figure 40.1Bi) are bonded to the teeth, using the acid-etch technique, or welded onto bands which can then be cemented using glass ionomer cement. Some clinicians will band the molars for the application of headgear or because of the reduced risk of bond failure and bond all other teeth. **Separators** are often placed 5–7 days before band placement to create space between the interproximal contacts to allow band placement.

Brackets systems can be manufactured from a number of different materials (e.g. stainless steel, ceramic), have different prescriptions for the final intended tooth position (e.g Andrews, Roth) and have many designs (e.g. ligating, self-ligating). The slot of the bracket has a rectangular shape in cross-section and is precisely cut to specific dimensions. The tip and inclination of the slot determines the final tooth position (Figure 40.1A). As the inclination and tip are calculated relative to the midpoint of the labial surface of the crown, it is essential that the bracket is positioned on this point, and parallel to the long axis of the tooth, to enable correct tooth positioning.

Archwires apply the active force to move teeth to their desired position (Figure 40.1Bii). They are constructed from various materials (e.g. stainless steel, nickel–titanium), have different cross-sectional shapes (round or rectangular) and have a large range of diameters. As the archwire is formed into a pre-determined archform, it will tend to move the teeth to this position unless the proportional limit of the wire is exceeded (Figure 40.1C).

During the early stages of treatment, flexible round wires are often used to deliver light forces and begin alignment. As the teeth progressively become straighter, stiffer rectangular wires can be used to correct tooth inclination, level the curve of Spee and provide a rigid guide for bodily tooth movement and space closure. Archwires are commonly held into the bracket slot using **elastomeric modules** (Figure 40.1Biii), which may be coloured, or stainless steel ligatures.

During treatment, archwires may protrude excessively from the most distal bracket and cause soft tissue trauma. These long 'distal ends' can be easily cut using specially designed pliers (distal-end cutters) that securely hold the excess wire to allow safe retrieval from the mouth.

Auxillaries are used to apply active forces for space opening or closure. Elastic materials can be used for intra-arch (intra-maxillary) space closure, and springs constructed from stainless steel or nickel titanium can be used for space opening (Figure 40.1D).

Stages of orthodontic treatment

For the purpose of learning, fixed appliance treatment can be subdivided into a number of stages. It is important to note that in a number of cases, the mechanical stages may overlap:
- Diagnosis and treatment planning (see Chapter 11);
- Anchorage control (see Chapter 37);
- Levelling and aligning;
- Overbite reduction (see Chapter 27);
- Overjet correction and space closure;
- Finishing;
- Retention (see Chapter 41).

Alignment refers to the correction of rotations, tip and inclination whereas **levelling** refers to the alignment of the bracket slots in the vertical plane. Levelling and alignment commences with the use of flexible aligning wires, which can be fully engaged into the bracket slot, and is complete when a large rectangular stainless steel wire (usually of 0.019×0.025 inch dimensions) lies passively within the bracket slot.

A deep **overbite** must be reduced before the incisors can be placed into a Class I relationship. For example, in a Class II case with a deep overbite, if the incisors are retracted without reducing the overbite, the lower incisal edges will clash with the cingulum of the upper incisors and prevent their retraction.

Overjet correction and space closure is undertaken in large rectangular wires which control the inclination of teeth. Space closing forces can be applied with intramaxillary and intermaxillary traction. It is important to reassess anchorage requirements before commencing space closure.

Common **finishing** procedures include adjustments to inclination and tip, centreline correction and occlusal settling. Final tip and inclination adjustments can be made by placing bends into the archwire or by repositioning incorrectly placed brackets. Centreline correction and settling is often undertaken using intermaxillary elastics.

Problems encountered during fixed appliance treatment

A number of risks of orthodontic treatment were outlined in Chapter 12. This section will concentrate on problems that may be encountered during fixed appliance treatment:

- There is large individual variation in the intensity of **pain** experienced by patients during fixed appliance treatment. Most will experience some pain that is caused by a localised inflammatory reaction around the tooth socket (see Chapter 35). Pain is commonly encountered following the placement of separators and after fixed appliance adjustments. It usually starts within a few hours of such a procedure, increases over the next 24 hours and decreases to baseline levels within 5–7 days. It may show diurnal variation with greatest intensity in the evening and night. Non-steroidal anti-inflammatory analgesics can be used in low doses, if necessary, to improve patient comfort.

- **Tooth mobility** is a normal phenomenon during tooth movement caused by disruption and an increased width of the periodontal ligament (see Chapter 35). Teeth with premature contacts may experience greater mobility, as can teeth on which excessive orthodontic forces are placed. In the majority of cases, the patient will just require reassurance if they are concerned about increased mobility, however, if the mobility is severe it may be worth taking a periapical radiograph to rule out severe root resorption (Figure 12.1C) or alveolar bone loss.

- **Mucosal trauma** is a common phenomenon during fixed appliance treatment. In the majority of cases a protruding wire is often the cause and is easy to deal with. Some patients may have exaggerated hyperplastic mucosal reactions to mild irritation caused by appliances rubbing on the mucosa. **Orthodontic wax** can be used to cushion the effects of appliance components.

- **Brackets may often debond** during a course of fixed appliance treatment. Patients should be advised to immediately see their orthodontist as a loss of control of debonded teeth and unwanted tooth movement may prolong treatment. Teeth with poorly developed enamel and a diet consisting of hard food predispose to multiple bracket failures.

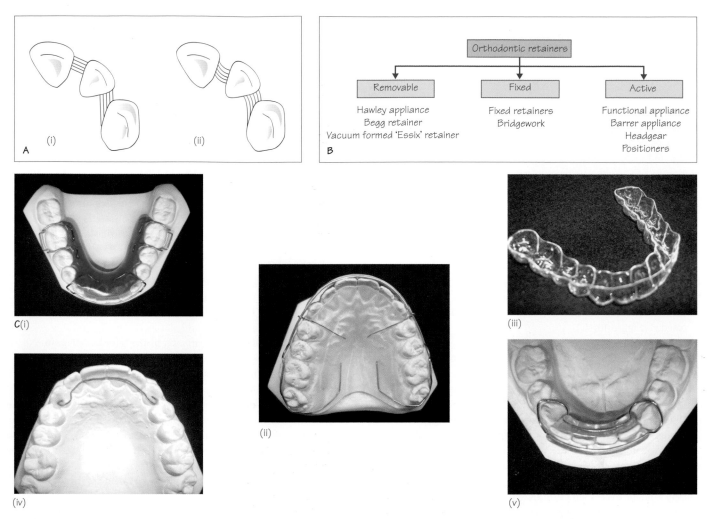

Figure 41.1 (**A**) (i) The transseptal fibres (shown in red) are an important cause of relapse of derotated teeth because of the long interval required for the fibres to reorganise following tooth movement. (ii) Derotation results in stretching of the fibres with generation of forces of elastic recoil. (**B**) A classification for orthodontic retainers. (**C**) Examples of orthodontic retainers: (i) Hawley retainer, (ii) Begg retainer, (iii) vacuum formed Essix-type retainer, (iv) fixed retainer and (v) Barrer spring retainer.

Orthodontic relapse is the term given when features of the original malocclusion return following the active phase of treatment. Retention is the phase of treatment following active tooth movement that is aimed at stabilising corrected intra-arch and inter-arch relationships. Retention should be planned during the treatment planning stage and discussed in detail as part of **informed consent**.

Orthodontic stability

Poor stability may occur for a number of reasons following treatment including:
- periodontal recovery;
- soft tissue imbalance;
- skeletal growth.

Orthodontic tooth movement results in disruption of the **periodontal and gingival** structures. Because these tissues are slow to remodel following orthodontic tooth movement, residual tension within the periodontal ligament and gingival fibres results in elastic recoil which moves teeth towards their pre-treatment position. To prevent relapse it is important to maintain the corrected positions until reorganisation is complete. Following appliance removal it takes approximately 3–4 months for the principal periodontal fibres, 4–6 months for the gingival fibres and 1 year for the transseptal fibres to reorganise if subjected to normal masticatory loading. Because of slow reorganisation of the **transseptal fibres**, derotated teeth are particularly prone to relapse (Figure 41.1A) and consideration should be given to long-term retention for severe rotations. **Pericision** may help to reduce the relapse of derotated teeth in the short term, however, the long-term benefits are questionable. This procedure involves surgically cutting the disrupted transseptal fibres by making a gingival crevicular incision under local anaesthesia following alignment.

If teeth are moved into an inherently unstable position during treatment, pressure from the **soft tissues**, such as the lips, cheeks and tongue, may result in relapse. This may occur if the lower incisors are excessively (>2 mm) advanced/proclined, if the dental arches are expanded out of soft tissue balance, and if the upper incisors are not controlled by the lower lip following incisor retraction (Class II cases). If such movements are undertaken intentionally, long-term retention should be planned at the treatment planning stage and discussed as part of informed consent.

The **skeletal growth** pattern existing before orthodontic treatment is likely to continue following appliance removal. This can result in a change in both inter-arch and intra-arch relationships. Vertical growth continues after the cessation of anteroposterior (AP) and transverse growth. Therefore, relapse in the vertical inter-arch relationship is more likely followed by anteroposterior and transverse changes. Unfavourable growth can result in a relapse of overbite and overjet correction.

Skeletal growth is also thought to contribute to **late lower incisor crowding** into middle age. Research clearly shows that the likelihood of maintaining acceptable lower incisor alignment in the long-term is extremely low (<30%) in orthodontically treated and untreated subjects. Continuing **differential mandibular growth** into adulthood (see Chapter 5) is likely to contribute to these changes as the lower incisors have to retrocline to compensate for this growth. Retroclination results in a decrease in arch circumference and crowding.

Extremes of **mandibular growth rotation**, both in a clockwise or anti-clockwise direction, also contributes to late lower incisor crowding (see Chapter 5). Other predisposing factors may include periodontal disease and soft tissue maturational changes that may alter the position of soft tissue balance. It is likely that the role of **third molars** in contributing to late lower incisor crowding has been overstated in the past as current evidence suggests no causal link.

Planning retention

As mentioned above, retention should be considered during the treatment planning stages. Most cases, with few exceptions, benefit from a period of retention. It is also important to follow certain orthodontic principles whilst undertaking treatment to maximise post-treatment stability: (a) maintaining the lower archform, (b) maintaining the AP position of the lower incisors, (c) retracting the upper incisors behind the lower lip in Class II cases, (d) correcting the inter-incisal angle following deep bite correction and (e) achieving good intercuspation (e.g. following crossbite correction).

The majority of patients completing fixed appliance treatment will benefit from **long-term retention** to minimise relapse and late lower incisor crowding. There are no current evidence-based guidelines on the ideal retention regimen. The author currently advises all patients to wear removable retainers every night for the first year and to cut down gradually to 2–3 nights/week indefinitely if long-term alignment is to be guaranteed.

Permanent retention should be planned in cases where the lower incisors have been proclined, large spaces have been closed, impacted canines have been aligned, severe rotations have been corrected and where there has been previous periodontal disease. Permanent retention can be effectively achieved with fixed retainers.

Retention appliances

A simple classification of orthodontic retainers is outlined in Figure 41.1B. Retainers can be classified according to whether they are removable, fixed or active. **Removable** retainers have the advantage that they are removable for oral hygiene measures, however, adequate wear is dependent on good compliance. **Fixed** retainers have the disadvantage of impeding oral hygiene, but are not dependent on patient compliance for wear. **Active** retainers are removable retainers that actively maintain inter-arch relationships during post-treatment growth or actively correct minor irregularities in tooth position (e.g. Barrer appliance).

The classic **Hawley appliance** consists of an acrylic baseplate with Adams clasps placed on the first molars and a labial bow with U-loops (Figure 41.1Ci). It can be used in both the upper and lower arches and has the advantage of being durable. Modifications exist including use of a labial bow with acrylic to maintain correction of rotations, a reverse U-loop to improve canine control, and a labial bow soldered to the bridge of the Adam clasps to minimise wirework crossing the occlusion and facilitate occlusal settling. The baseplate can be modified into a U-shape to minimise palatal coverage and improve comfort and speech. An anterior bite plane can be included for maintenance of deep bite correction. The **Begg retainer** (Figure 41.1Cii) is a modified version of the Hawley retainer that does not incorporate Adams clasps and therefore allows greater molar settling.

Vacuum formed thermoplastic retainers (e.g. the Essix appliance) are popular because of their high patient acceptability, good aesthetics (Figure 41.1Ciii), ease of manufacture and low cost. These retainers are not as durable as Hawley-type retainers.

Fixed retainers are commonly constructed from 0.0175-inch diameter multi-strand stainless steel wire that can be bonded with composite resin to the lingual surfaces of the lower incisors and canines. They can also be used in the upper arch to maintain diastema closure and correction of severe rotations, and also after alignment of impacted canines (Figure 41.1Civ). Fixed retainers can be constructed at the chairside or in the laboratory. Their main advantage is that they are not dependent on patient compliance for wear. Disadvantages include difficulty with oral hygiene, localised relapse and decalcification following partial debond. Bonded retainers should be supplemented with removable retainers, which can be worn if breakages occur.

Active retainers can be used to correct and maintain inter-arch and intra-arch dental relationships. A functional appliance can be used for the remainder of the growth period following Class II and Class III correction. The appliance is worn on a night-only basis and helps to maintain alignment as well as incisor correction. High-pull headgear can also be incorporated into an upper appliance to help control vertical maxillary growth in Class II cases with an increased vertical dimension.

The **Barrer spring retainer** (Figure 41.1Cv) is an active retainer that can be used to correct minor irregularities in incisor alignment. The teeth are sectioned and aligned on a working model and the appliance is constructed to the corrected position. When it is inserted into the mouth an active force is placed onto the teeth to be repositioned until tooth movement is complete. Interproximal enamel reduction may be necessary to provide space for alignment.

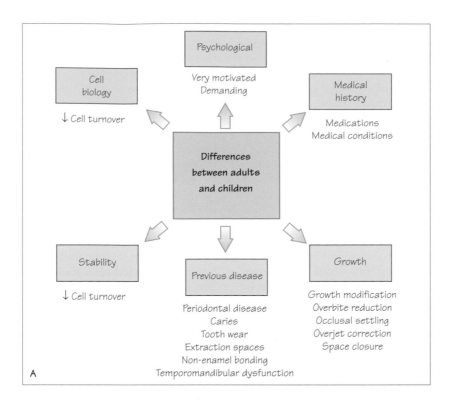

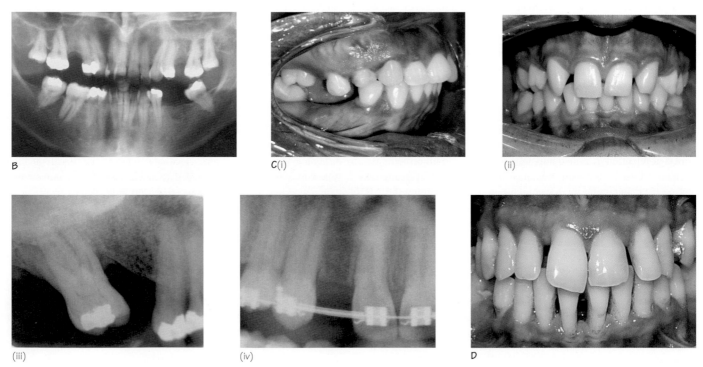

Figure 42.1 (**A**) The differences between treating adults and children. (**B**) Previous dental disease can complicate orthodontic management as in this patient who has a heavily restored dentition, periodontal disease and previous tooth loss. (**C**) Orthodontics can be used to facilitate restorative treatment: (i) Intrusion of over-erupted upper right first premolar, (ii) re-creation of space for missing lateral incisors, (iii) uprighting of potential bridge abutments and (iv) root paralleling and separation for the placement of implants. (**D**) Periodontal destruction predisposes to pathological tooth migration such as spacing, extrusion and rotation of affected teeth.

The demand for adult orthodontics has increased dramatically over the past two decades. This is due to a number of factors including a greater awareness of the importance of an aesthetic smile, an appreciation of how orthodontics can facilitate restorative dentistry and the introduction of more aesthetically pleasing and socially acceptable appliances. Orthodontic treatment in adults may be provided to improve aesthetics, function and/or facilitate restorative treatment.

Differences between treating adults and children

The differences between treating adults and children are summarised in Figure 42.1A.

Psychologically, adults have often made a conscious effort to seek orthodontic care and are often more clear about what they would like to achieve. They may be keen to have aesthetically appearing appliances for social or professional reasons. A major benefit of treating adults is that they can be extremely motivated and compliant with instructions (e.g. oral hygiene, elastic wear).

Unlike the majority of children, adult patients may have a complicated **medical history**. The actual condition, or the medications that are used for its treatment, can alter the way in which care is delivered.

A major difference between treating adults and children is the lack of **facial growth** in older patients. Favourable facial growth in children can facilitate space closure, overjet (e.g. functional appliances) and overbite (e.g. biteplanes) reduction. As the dentition erupts to compensate for vertical skeletal growth, there is mesial migration that aids space closure. A lack of growth in adults can complicate the above mentioned movements and increase anchorage requirements. The threshold for the management of skeletal discrepancies with orthognathic surgery is lower in adults than children as a result of these differences.

Adult patients have often been affected by a lifetime of **dental disease** that can complicate their orthodontic management. They may have had periodontal disease, caries and tooth surface loss (Figure 42.1B). Heavily broken down teeth may have been restored with crowns which can complicate bonding of orthodontic brackets. The presence of heavily restored teeth may necessitate non-ideal extraction patterns (e.g. extraction of first molars) which can complicate anchorage management especially as adults are less likely to accept headgear. If there have been previous extractions the alveolar ridge may have atrophied and make space closure impossible. Space for the relief of mild crowding can be created by interproximal enamel reduction and reduction of large mesial and distal restorations. Interproximal enamel reduction is more feasible in adults than children due to the presence of greater amounts of secondary dentine, however, care needs to be taken when assessing enamel thickness, as this may have been reduced by tooth surface loss.

Due to reduced **cellular activity**, the time taken to initiate tooth movement is often prolonged in adults, however, once commenced tooth movement occurs at a similar rate to children. Adults may experience more **pain** following archwire adjustments and it may be wise to use lighter initial aligning forces. Adults may experience greater **root resorption** than younger patients due to reduced vascularity of the periodontal ligament. The **periodontal fibres** in adult patients may not adapt to altered tooth positions as quickly as in children, which may mean adoption of stricter retention regimens.

Orthodontics to facilitate restorative treatment

Orthodontics is being increasingly used to facilitate prosthodontic treatment (Figure 42.1C). It can help improve the aesthetics and survival of restorations. The treatment for patients attending for such care should be planned jointly by the orthodontist and prosthodontist. Examples of tooth movements that can facilitate restorative treatment include:

• **Space redistribution** which can help improve the final aesthetic outcome and decrease the failure of restorations by reducing pontic spans.
• **Root paralleling** and separation can facilitate implant placement.
• **Overbite reduction** can help improve the lifetime of anterior restorations.
• **Intrusion** of over-erupted teeth to provide space for restorative treatment.
• **Extrusion** of fractured teeth for supra-gingival margin placement.
• **Uprighting** of tilted abutment teeth.

The periodontally compromised patient

Attachment loss can result in **pathological tooth migration** particularly when the soft tissues are unfavourable and occlusal loads are high. Tooth movements that occur, and particularly affect the incisors, include tipping, rotation, over-eruption and spacing (Figure 42.1D).

With effective plaque and disease control, teeth with reduced periodontal support can undergo successful tooth movement without further compromising their periodontal health. Treatment undertaken in the presence of inflammatory disease can accelerate attachment loss and predisposes to acute inflammatory episodes.

During treatment it is essential that oral hygiene is excellent and patients should have 3-monthly hygiene visits to facilitate this. Orthodontic appliances can be made less plaque retentive by using mini-brackets, bonded attachments rather than bands, removal of excess composite adhesive and avoiding elastomeric modules which swell in the mouth and are plaque retentive.

Anchorage management may be more difficult in both the anteroposterior and vertical dimension as molar teeth with reduced attachment levels offer less resistance to unwanted tooth movement. It is important to minimise any extrusion of molars as this may further reduce attachment levels, and extrusive movement is unstable. It is also necessary to use light forces as teeth affected by periodontal disease are more likely to tip, as the centre of tooth resistance moves apically with bone loss (see Chapter 36), and the risk of root resorption is greater due to a reduced root surface area.

Following treatment patients will require **permanent retention** either with fixed or removable retainers (Figure 41.1A). Periodontally compromised teeth are prone to relapse.

Table 43.1 Examples of orthognathic surgical procedures.

Surgical procedure	Notes
Maxillary	
Le Fort 1	Addresses AP and vertical maxillary discrepancies
Le Fort 2	Addresses deficiency of the naso-maxillary complex
Le Fort 3	Addresses deficiency of the naso-maxillary complex and zygoma
Wassermund	An anterior maxillary segmental osteotomy for setbacks and setdowns
Mandibular	
BSSO	For anterior-posterior and asymmetrical mandibular movements
Genioplasty	To move the chin point in three dimensions
Total subapical osteotomy	For correction of dento-alveolar retrusion

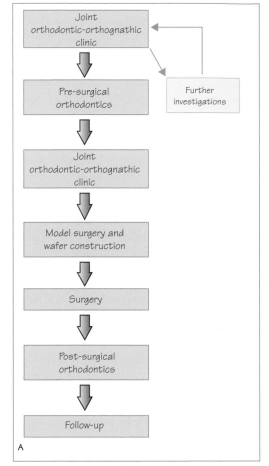

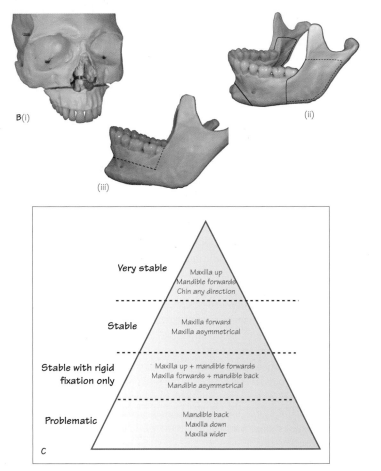

Figure 43.1 (**A**) Outline of the patient journey through joint orthodontic-orthognathic surgical treatment. (**B**) Surgical anatomy (i) Le Fort 1 osteotomy, (ii) Genioplasty (red line) and BSSO osteotomy, and (iii) total subapical osteotomy. (**C**) The hierachy of surgical stability. The surgical procedures progressively become less stable as one moves down the list.

Orthodontics in combination with orthognathic surgery is undertaken for the comprehensive management of malocclusion associated with severe skeletal discrepancies in the anteroposterior (AP), vertical and transverse dimensions. This form of treatment is normally undertaken at the end of growth to improve post-treatment stability.

Successful management requires a **multidisciplinary team** approach involving an orthodontist, oral and maxillofacial surgeon, liaison psychiatrist, general dental practitioner, clinic co-ordinator, technician and sometimes a prosthodontist. Figure 43.1A outlines the patient journey

during this form of treatment. The time period between the first multidisciplinary clinic appointment to the end of treatment is usually 2.5–3 years.

Joint orthodontic-orthognathic clinic

Full records, including study models, radiographs and photographs, should be available for the consultation. The purpose of the first joint orthodontic-orthognathic appointment is to introduce the patient to the multidisciplinary team, identify their main concerns, discuss the feasibility of treatment and obtain informed consent (**risk–benefit analysis**). Understanding and addressing the patient's main concerns is essential for a successful treatment outcome. Computerised prediction software (e.g. Dolphin) is available to allow visualisation of proposed treatment changes.

At the end of this consultation, there should be a clear idea of the orthodontic and surgical treatment plan unless further information is required. This may involve assessment by the liaison psychiatrist, advanced imaging studies (e.g. computed tomography (CT) scans in those with complex asymmetries) or investigations to assess the long-term prognosis of individual teeth.

Pre-surgical orthodontics

Pre-surgical orthodontics, undertaken with **fixed appliances**, has the following aims:

- alignment;
- decompensation of incisor inclinations;
- arch co-ordination;
- creation of space for interdental osteotomy cuts;
- facilitation of the placement of temporary intermaxillary fixation during surgery.

It is necessary to **decompensate** the incisor inclinations to allow the necessary surgical movements and to achieve a satisfactory occlusion following surgery. In Class II cases this will often involve retroclination of the lower incisors, and in Class III cases it will involve retroclination of the upper and proclination of the lower incisors. It is important to undertake a space analysis as extractions may be required especially in those cases requiring significant incisor retraction. **Anchorage** may be reinforced with intermaxillary traction. Class II elastics are usually used in skeletal III cases and Class III elastics in skeletal II cases. Decompensation will unmask the original malocclusion and make the patient look worse before surgery is undertaken. It is important that the patient is warned about this before commencing treatment.

Arch co-ordination refers to co-ordinating the widths of the dental arches so that there is a normal transverse relationship following AP jaw movements. Treatment will often involve upper arch expansion in Class II and III cases using archwires or a quad helix appliance (Figure 30.1C). In those cases with significant transverse deficiencies, surgical expansion maybe the only alternative.

In cases that require segmental jaw surgery, it is necessary to **create space** between the roots of teeth to enable surgical cuts to be made without damaging dental structures. A segmental surgical approach may be required in patients with transverse maxillary deficiency, where upper arch expansion is required, and in those with an anterior open bite where there is a step in the maxillary occlusal plane.

At the end of pre-surgical orthodontics it is important to securely tie passive 0.019″ × 0.025″ stainless steel archwires by using steel ligatures and fix hooks onto the archwire that enable placement of temporary intermaxillary fixation during surgery. **Full records** should be taken at the end of pre-surgical orthodontics.

Joint orthodontic-orthognathic clinic

At the end of pre-surgical orthodontics, the patients should be reassessed on the joint clinic to finalise the surgical movements. This also provides a valuable opportunity for members of the multidisciplinary team to co-ordinate the final stages of treatment (e.g. wafer construction).

Model surgery and wafer construction

Model surgery, using study models mounted on a **semi-adjustable articulator**, is undertaken in those cases requiring maxillary surgery. It allows an assessment of the effects of maxillary surgery on mandibular position (i.e. autorotation) and facilitates construction of surgical wafers. In cases requiring bimaxillary surgery, two surgical wafers have to be constructed. The first, or intermediary, wafer guides positioning of the maxilla in relation to the pre-surgical mandibular position. The second, or final, wafer positions the mandible in relation to the new maxillary position. In cases involving mandibular surgery alone, only one surgical wafer is required that guides positioning of the mandible in relation to the maxilla.

Surgery

Table 43.1 and Figure 43.1B outline some of the surgical procedures. In cases requiring bimaxillary surgery, it is usual to reposition the maxilla first (using the first or intermediary wafer) and then position the mandible (using the second or final wafer) in relation to the corrected maxillary position. Temporary intermaxillary fixation, using elastics running between archwire hooks, can be used to stabilise jaw position during fixation.

For maxillary surgery, an incision is made around the full length of the sulcus to gain access to the underlying bone. The most common form of maxillary surgery is the Le Fort 1 osteotomy to advance and/or vertically reposition the maxilla. The maxilla may be impacted posteriorly to reduce the lower anterior facial height and increase the overbite. The anterior vertical maxillary position is determined by the need to have 2–4 mm of incisor show at rest.

The most commonly performed mandibular procedure is the bilateral sagittal split osteotomy (BSSO) which can be undertaken using a posteriorly based intra-oral incision. The BSSO can be used to advance, setback or asymmetrically reposition the mandible. The third molars are commonly removed at least 6 months before the procedure to facilitate the osteotomy. A major risk of the BSSO is damage to the inferior dental nerve which can result in permanent (5–10% of cases) paraesthesia.

Osteotomies are **rigidly fixated** using titanium plates and screws which have reduced the necessity for post-surgical intermaxillary fixation and improve the stability of final surgery. There is a small risk of post-operative infection associated with plating.

Post-surgical orthodontics

Some surgeons prefer to leave the second (final) wafer *in situ* following surgery to provide occlusal contacts which direct the mandible into its correct position. This may be unnecessary in those cases where there is a good post-surgical occlusion. Intermaxillary elastics can be used in the immediate post-surgical period to help guide mandibular position as proprioception is often reduced.

The aims of post-surgical orthodontics is to produce a well-intercuspated occlusion which will help to improve the stability of surgery. This may involve the use of intermaxillary elastics and the fine tuning of arch co-ordination. Post-surgical orthodontics should take no longer than 6 months in the average case. Following debond, patients should be provided with upper and lower retainers.

Recall

Patients should be reviewed on an annual basis following surgery for up to 5 years. This provides an opportunity to identify complications and audit treatment outcomes. Complications following surgery include patient dissatisfaction with treatment, paraesthesia in the distribution of the inferior dental nerve, infection of bone plates and relapse. Figure 43.1C outlines the hierarchy of surgical stability.

44 Cleft lip and palate

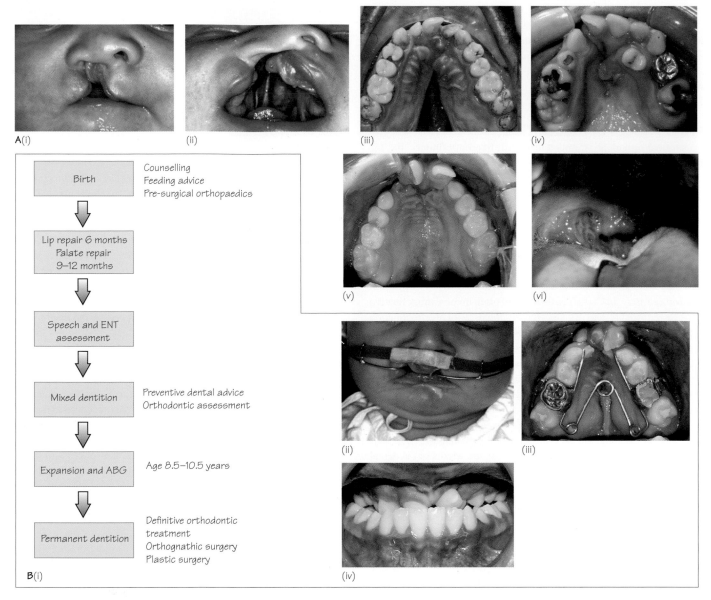

Table 44.1 A simplified version of the Kernahan and Stark classification of cleft lip and palate.

Clefts of the primary palate	Clefts of the secondary palate	Clefts of the primary and secondary palate
Unilateral (left or right)	Complete	Unilateral (left or right)
Complete	Incomplete	Complete
Incomplete	Submucous	Incomplete
Bilateral		Bilateral
Complete		Complete
Incomplete		Incomplete

Figure 44.1 (**A**) Examples of cleft lip and palate: (i–iii) unilateral complete cleft of the lip and palate (primary and secondary) (iv) unilateral complete cleft of the lip and primary palate, (v) bilateral complete cleft of the lip and primary palate, and (vi) a bifid uvula which may suggest a submucous cleft. (**B**) (i) Care pathway for the management of cleft lip and palate, (ii) pre-surgical orthopaedics with lip strapping, (iii) a tri-helix appliance used to achieve expansion before alveolar bone grafting (ABG), and (iv) a Class III relationship that is often evident and requires joint orthodontic-orthognathic treatment.

Cleft lip and palate (CLP) is the most common congenital craniofacial deformity. Its incidence varies according to the ethnic group studied: American Indians (1/300 live births) > Japanese (1/400) > Chinese (1/500) > Caucasians (1/600) > black people (1/2500). Cleft lip (CL) ± cleft palate (CL(P)), forms a separate entity from isolated clefts of the secondary palate (CP), with a difference in incidence, gender bias and genetic contribution. CL(P) is approximately twice as common in males as females, whereas, isolated CP is twice as common in females.

Aetiology

CL arises from failure of fusion (at 7 weeks *in utero*) between the medial nasal, lateral nasal and maxillary swellings. CP arises from failure of fusion (8–9 weeks *in utero*) of the lateral palatal swellings.

CLP may be isolated or as part of a syndrome. The aetiology of isolated CLP is **multifactorial** with both genetic and environmental influences. There is a family history of CL(P) in approximately 40% of individuals whereas the corresponding figure in CP is 20%. Environmental risk factors include maternal alcohol intake, smoking and phenytoin intake. Folic acid may have a protective effect. Many conditions can be associated with CP including Pierre–Robin sequence, hemifacial microsomia, Treacher Collins syndrome and Stickler syndrome.

Classification of CLP

The severity of a cleft can vary from a mild deformity (submucous cleft, *forme fruste* of the lip) to a complete bilateral CLP. Many classifications exist, a popular one is that of Kernahan and Stark (Table 44.1). In this classification, primary palate refers to the lip, alveolus and palate anterior to the incisive foramen. A complete cleft of the primary palate will involve the full thickness of these structures. Figure 44.1A shows clinical examples of various types of cleft.

Clinical problems in CLP

Clinical problems depend on the severity and location of the cleft. These include:
- **Feeding** difficulty due to communication between the oral and nasal cavities.
- **Hearing** problems secondary to poor middle ear drainage due to Eustachian tube dysfunction.
- **Speech** defects due to velopharyngeal incompetence and secondarily to poor hearing.
- **Dental anomalies** include: (a) hypodontia (50% have a missing lateral incisor on the cleft side), (b) supernumerary or supplemental lateral incisors, (c) maxillary canine impaction (×10 risk), (d) delayed dental development, (d) hypoplastic teeth, (e) microdontia and (f) impaction of first permanent molars.
- **Malocclusion** including anterior and posterior crossbites.
- **Deficient maxillary growth** related to scarring of the maxilla following palate repair.
- **Low self-esteem**.

Treatment

The treatment of CLP involves a **multidisciplinary approach** by a dedicated cleft lip and palate team. An example of a care pathway is given in Figure 44.1Bi.

At the time of birth the parents should receive **counselling** and the contact details of a support group, e.g. Cleft Lip and Palate Association (CLAPA). Special **feeding** bottles (e.g. Haberman feeder), which eject fluid without the infant having to generate negative intra-oral pressure, can be helpful if breast feeding is unsuccessful.

Presurgical orthopaedics, with a maxillary removable appliance, can be used to encourage lateral palatal shelf growth by stopping the tongue from sitting within the cleft site. Such plates, used up to the time of palatal surgery, facilitate palate repair by approximating the cleft segments. Extra-oral lip strapping can be used in bilateral CLP to control growth of the premaxilla which facilitates lip closure (Figure 44.1Bii).

The surgical protocol for CLP can vary between teams due to the lack of evidence to support any one protocol. Many undertake **lip repair** at 6 months by re-alignment of muscle fibres, to encourage normal function, and skin closure. **Palatal repair** is undertaken at 9–12 months to encourage development of normal speech. Dissection should be minimal to limit scarring that may hinder future maxillary growth.

As the deciduous teeth erupt, **preventive dental advice** (oral hygiene, dietary and use of fluorides) is important to establish good dental health. A **speech assessment** should be undertaken by 2 years to detect any speech abnormality. An **ENT opinion**, to assess hearing, can also be useful as patients often have middle ear drainage problems.

At 6–8 years **psychological support** maybe required as children start to notice that they are different and may be teased. Preventive dental advice should continue into the mixed dentition where fissure sealing may be helpful. A **full orthodontic assessment** is also important at this stage. Removable/fixed appliances can be used to correct anterior crossbites in concerned patients. Care should be taken not to move teeth towards the cleft as the lack of bone may cause root exposure.

Alevolar bone grafting (ABG) is usually undertaken between 8.5–10.5 years when the root of the maxillary canine is half to two-thirds formed. The role of ABG is to provide bone, usually taken from the iliac crest, for canine eruption, offer bony support to teeth on either side of the cleft, close residual palatal fistulae and provide nasal support. **Expansion**, with a quad/tri-helix (Figure 44.1Biii), is often necessary before bone grafting to expand the collapsed cleft segment and improve access to the site. Fixed appliances should be used to stabilise the mobile premaxilla in bilateral complete CLP prior to ABG.

Once in the permanent dentition, **definitive orthodontic treatment** can be undertaken. Patients often have a Class III malocclusion due to deficient maxillary growth (Figure 44.1Biv). The tight cleft lip and a lack of overbite may potentiate relapse following treatment. Where there is a severe skeletal discrepancy an **orthognathic approach**, almost certainly involving maxillary advancement, may be undertaken near the completion of growth. This should be planned with care because it may further compromise speech, by effecting velopharyngeal function, and there is a high risk of relapse. **Distraction osteogenesis** (see Glossary) may help to reduce these complications as it produces skeletal change by slow movement that produces gradual stretching of the soft tissues.

The **replacement of missing teeth** with implants can also be undertaken at the end of growth assuming there is adequate bone volume at the site of implant placement.

Patients may have a number of **plastic surgery** procedures to improve nasal aesthetics, lip revision and close residual palatal fistulae during the CLP care pathway.

Appendix 1 The Index of Orthodontic Treatment Need (IOTN)

Dental Health Component of IOTN

GRADE 5 (Need treatment)

5.i   Impeded eruption of teeth (except for third molars) due to crowding, displacement, the presence of supernumerary teeth, retained deciduous teeth and any pathological cause.

5.h   Extensive hypodontia with restorative implications (more than 1 tooth missing in any quadrant) requiring pre-restorative orthodontics.

5.a   Increased overjet greater than 9 mm.

5.m   Reverse overjet greater than 3.5 mm with reported masticatory and speech difficulties.

5.p   Defects of cleft lip and palate and other craniofacial anomalies.

5.s   Submerged deciduous teeth.

GRADE 4 (Need treatment)

4.h   Less extensive hypodontia requiring prerestorative orthodontics or orthodontic space closure to obviate the need for a prosthesis.

4.a   Increased overjet greater than 6 mm but less than or equal to 9 mm.

4.b   Reverse overjet greater than 3.5 mm with no masticatory or speech difficulties.

4.m   Reverse overjet greater than 1 mm but less than 3.5 mm with recorded masticatory and speech difficulties.

4.c   Anterior or posterior crossbites with greater than 2 mm discrepancy between retruded contact position and intercuspal position.

4.l   Posterior lingual crossbite with no functional occlusal contact in one or both buccal segments.

4.d   Severe contact point displacements greater than 4 mm.

4.e   Extreme lateral or anterior open bites greater than 4 mm.

4.f   Increased and complete overbite with gingival or palatal trauma.

4.t   Partially erupted teeth, tipped and impacted against adjacent teeth.

4.x   Presence of supernumerary teeth.

GRADE 3 (Borderline need)

3.a   Increased overjet greater than 3.5 mm but less than or equal to 6 mm with incompetent lips.

3.b   Reverse overjet greater than 1 mm but less than or equal to 3.5 mm.

3.c   Anterior or posterior crossbites with greater than 1 mm but less than or equal to 2 mm discrepancy between retruded contact position and intercuspal position.

3.d   Contact point displacements greater than 2 mm but less than or equal to 4 mm.

3.e   Lateral or anterior open bite greater than 2 mm but less than or equal to 4 mm.

3.f   Deep overbite complete on gingival or palatal tissues but no trauma.

GRADE 2 (Little)

2.a   Increased overjet greater than 3.5 mm but less than or equal to 6 mm with competent lips.

2.b   Reverse overjet greater than 0 mm but less than or equal to 1 mm.

2.c   Anterior or posterior crossbite with less than or equal to 1 mm discrepancy between retruded contact position and intercuspal position.

2.d   Contact point displacements greater than 1 mm but less than or equal to 2 mm.

2.e   Anterior or posterior openbite greater than 1 mm but less than or equal to 2 mm.

2.f   Increased overbite greater than or equal 3.5 mm without gingival contact.

2.g   Pre-normal or post-normal occlusions with no other anomalies (includes up to half a unit discrepancy).

GRADE 1 (None)

1.   Extremely minor maloccusions including contact point displacements less than 1 mm.

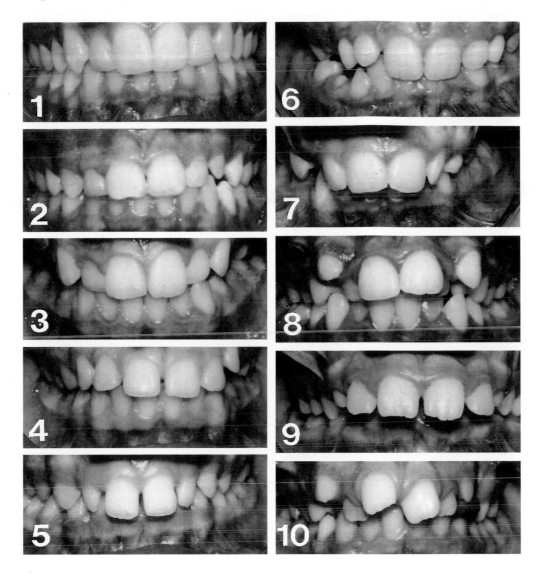

Appendix 2 Commonly used cephalometric points and reference lines

A-point (A) — The deepest point in the concavity between ANS and the upper incisor alveolar crest. This point signifies the anterior limit of the maxilla but has the drawback that its position can be altered by anteroposterior (AP) movement of the upper incisors.

Anterior nasal spine (ANS) — The tip of the anterior nasal spine.

B-point (B) — The deepest point in the concavity between pogonion and the lower incisor alveolar crest. This position of this point is affected by AP movement of the lower incisors.

Glabella — The most prominent anterior point on the forehead.

Gnathion — The most anterior inferior point of the bony outline of the chin.

Gonion (Go) — The most posterior inferior point on the angle of the mandible. If the images of the mandibular angle are not superimposed, this suggests a mandibular asymmetry, and an average outline should be contructed to identify gonion.

Menton (Me) — The lowest point on the bony outline of the mandibular symphysis.

Nasion (N) — The most anterior point on the frontonasal suture representing the anterior limit of the cranial base.

Orbitale (Or) — The most anterior inferior point on the infra-orbital margin. If the images of the two orbits are not superimposed the average can be used.

Pogonion (Pog) — The most anterior point on the bony chin.

Porion (Po) — The uppermost point of the bony external auditory meatus which is usually level with the superior surface of the condyle. If the external meatus is obscured by the ear rods, the condyle can be used to locate its vertical position.

Posterior nasal spine (PNS) — The tip of the posterior nasal spine of the palatine bone. It may be obscured by the developing third molars in which case its position can be approximated to lie beneath the pterygomaxillary fissure.

Sella (S) — The midpoint of the sella turcica.

Soft tissue A-point — The most concave portion of the upper lip in the midline.

Soft tissue B-point — The most concave portion of the lower lip in the midline.

Soft tissue menton — The most inferior point of the chin in the midline.

Soft tissue nasion — The most concave aspect of the bridge of the nose in the midline.

Soft tissue pogonion — The most prominent point on the soft tissue chin in the midline.

S-N line — The line connecting sella and nasion and representing the cranial base.

Subnasale — The point at which the columella merges with the upper lip in the midline.

Frankfort plane — The line connecting porion and orbitale. The disadvantage of this plane is the difficulty in accurately locating Po and Or.

Mandibular plane — The line joining gonion and menton.

Maxillary plane — The line joining anterior nasal spine and posterior nasal spine.

Functional occlusal plane — A line drawn between the cusps of the molars and premolars.

Glossary of orthodontic terms

Adaptive swallowing pattern: A swallowing pattern that exists when a normal lip to lip anterior oral seal cannot be achieved.

Anchorage: The resistance to unwanted three-dimensional forces generated in reaction to the active components of an appliance.

Angle classification: A classification of malocclusion introduced by Edward Angle based on the anteroposterior relationship of the first permanent molars.

Angulation: The mesiodistal angulation of the long axis of a tooth in relationship to a line drawn perpendicular to the occlusal plane (compare with *inclination*).

Ankylosis: An abnormal fusion between two bones or between a tooth and bone.

Anodontia: The developmental absence of all primary and secondary teeth.

Anterior open bite: Where no vertical overlap exists between the maxillary and mandibular incisors when the molars are in occlusion.

Anterior oral seal: A seal produced between the lips, the lower lip and palate or the tongue and lips to prevent expulsion of a bolus during mastication.

Arch form: The shape of the mandibular or maxillary arch.

Archwire: A wire engaged into orthodontic brackets to provide the active forces for tooth movement and/or a stable platform for bodily tooth movement.

Autorotation: Rotation of the mandible around the condylar axis following vertical maxillary repositioning.

Balancing extraction: Extraction of a contralateral tooth during the mixed dentition to minimise a shift of the dental centreline (compare with *compensating extraction*).

Bilateral sagittal split osteotomy (BSSO): A surgical mandibular procedure, where the ramus is split parallel to the sagittal plane, commonly used to advance, setback and rotate the mandible.

Bimaxillary: Relating to both upper and lower dentoalveolar segments.

Bimaxillary protrusion: A term used to describe protrusion of the maxilla and mandible in relationship to the cranial base.

Bimaxillary retrusion: A term used to describe retrusion of the maxilla and mandible in relationship to the cranial base.

Bolton (tooth size) discrepancy: A mismatch between the sum of mesiodistal widths of the maxillary and mandibular dentition making it difficult to achieve an ideal occlusal fit.

Buccal segment: The canines, premolars and molars.

Camouflage (orthodontic): Occlusal compensation of mild/moderate skeletal discrepancies by orthodontic tooth movement.

Centric occlusion: The position of maximum intercuspation.

Centric relation: The relationship between the mandible and maxilla with the condyles in an unrestrained retruded position within the glenoid fossae.

Class I incisor relationship: A term used to describe a malocclusion where the lower incisor edges occlude on or directly beneath the cingulum plateau of the upper incisors (British Standards Institute classification).

Class II division 1 incisor relationship: A term used to describe a malocclusion where the lower incisor edges lie posterior to the cingulum plateau of the upper incisors, the overjet is increased and the upper central incisors are normally inclined or proclined (British Standards Institute classification).

Class II division 2 incisor relationship: A term used to describe a malocclusion where the lower incisal edges occlude posterior to the cingulum plateau of the upper incisors, and the upper central incisors are retroclined (British Standards Institute classification).

Class III incisor relationship: A term used to describe a malocclusion where two or more of the lower incisal edges occlude anterior to the cingulum plateau of the upper incisors (British Standards Institute classification).

Class II intermaxillary traction: Intermaxillary anchorage provided by placing elastics between the maxillary incisors and mandibular molars.

Class III intermaxillary traction: Intermaxillary anchorage provided by placing elastics between the maxillary molars and mandibular incisors.

Class I malocclusion (Angle classification): A malocclusion where the buccal groove of the mandibular first permanent molar occludes with the mesiobuccal cusp of the maxillary first molar.

Class II malocclusion (Angle classification): A malocclusion where the buccal groove of the mandibular first permanent molar occludes posterior to the mesiobuccal cusp of the maxillary first molar. A Class II division 1 malocclusion describes this relationship when the maxillary central incisors are proclined or normally inclined and the overjet is increased. A Class II division 2 malocclusion describes this relationship when the maxillary central incisors are retroclined.

Class III malocclusion (Angle classification): A malocclusion where the buccal groove of the mandibular first permanent molar occludes anterior to the mesiobuccal cusp of the maxillary first molar.

Compensating extraction: Extraction of an opposing tooth during the mixed dentition to prevent its over-eruption (compare to *balancing extraction*).

Competent lips: An anterior lip seal can be achieved with minimal muscular activity with the mandible in the rest position.

Complete overbite: The lower incisors occlude with the upper incisors or palatal mucosa when the teeth are in occlusion.

Couple: A pair of equal and opposite parallel forces applied to a body.

Crossbite: An abnormal relationship between occluding teeth in a buccolingual and/or labiolingual direction.

Curve of Spee: A convex curve, when viewed in the sagittal plane, produced by the curvature of the cusps and incisal edges of the mandibular teeth. The depth of the curve positively correlates with the depth of the overbite.

Decompensation: The removal of adaptive occlusal changes in the dentition which mask the severity of a skeletal discrepancy. It is undertaken prior to orthognathic surgery.

Dento-alveolar adaptation: The dynamic process of occlusal adaptation, produced by favourable soft tissues, which masks the severity of an underlying skeletal discrepancy in the anteroposterior, vertical or transverse dimension.

Dento-alveolar compensation: A static snapshot of occlusal adaptation, produced by favourable soft tissues, which masks the severity of a skeletal discrepancy in the anteroposterior, vertical or transverse dimension.

Deviation (mandibular): A sagittal movement of the mandible during closure from a habit posture into centric occlusion.

Diagnostic (Kesling) setup: A diagnostic laboratory procedure where the teeth are sectioned from a duplicate model and realigned into their desired position to study the occlusal outcome of a proposed treatment plan.

Diastema: A naturally occurring space between teeth.

Dilaceration: The presence of an abnormal bend or curve in the root or crown of a tooth commonly as a result of dental trauma.

Displacement (mandibular): A sagittal and/or lateral movement of the mandible on closing from centric relation into centric occlusion as a result of an occlusal interference.

Distraction osteogenesis: A surgical technique for lengthening bones, and their associated soft tissue envelope, involving corticotomy followed by gradual separation (distraction) of the bone segments (1 mm/day) and osseous infill.

Facemask: An extra-oral appliance, commonly used in Class III malocclusion, that uses anchorage from the chin and forehead in order to place anterior forces on the maxillary dentition and/or maxilla.

Fixed appliance: An appliance that is cemented or bonded onto the teeth and cannot be removed by the patient.

Functional appliance: A removable or fixed appliance, usually used in Class II malocclusion, which alters the posture of the mandible, causing stretching of the facial soft tissues, to produce a combination of dental and skeletal changes.

Functional matrix theory: A theory of facial growth suggesting that skeletal growth is determined by the functional spaces and soft tissues associated with any skeletal unit.

Frenum: A fold of mucous membrane and underlying fibrous tissue.

Genioplasty: An orthognathic procedure undertaken to reposition the bony chin point anteroposteriorly, vertically and/or transversely.

Growth rotation: A rotation of the core of the mandible and maxilla in relationship to the cranial base that occurs with normal growth. Growth rotations are commonly described as being clockwise (backwards) or anti-clockwise (forwards).

Headgear: An extra-oral appliance using cervical or cranial anchorage to apply forces to the teeth or jaws for tooth movement or growth modification, respectively.

Hyalinization: A term used to describe the loss of cells from an area as seen by light microscope.

Hypodontia: The developmental absence of one or more teeth excluding the third molars.

Impaction: Failure of a tooth to erupt due to insufficient space or an obstruction, ectopic positioning or pathology.

Imbrication: Overlapping of the incisors due to crowding.

Inclination: The labiolingual or buccolingual angulation of the long axis of a tooth in relationship to a line drawn perpendicular to the occlusal plane (compare to *angulation*).

Incompetent lips: Where excessive muscular activity is required to achieve an anterior lip seal with the mandible in the rest position.

Incomplete overbite: The lower incisors do not contact the uppers or the palatal mucosa when the teeth are in occlusion.

Informed consent: The process of providing the patient, or parent in the case of children, with relevant information regarding the treatment options, their relative advantages and disadvantages and the consequences of no treatment.

Infraocclusion: The positioning of a tooth below the occlusal plane.

Interference (occlusal): An occlusal contact occurring during mandibular closure from centric relation into centric occlusion that results in a mandibular displacement.

Intermaxillary: Between the dental arches.

Intermaxillary space: The space between the upper and lower dental arches with the mandible in the rest position.

Interproximal enamel reduction: The removal of interproximal enamel for space creation.

Intramaxillary: Within the same dental arch.

Labial segment: The incisor teeth.

Leeway space: The difference between the combined width of the deciduous canine, first and second molar in each quadrant and their successors.

Le Fort 1 osteotomy: A surgical maxillary procedure, in which the maxilla is osteotomised just above the tooth apices, used to advance or vertically reposition the maxilla.

Levelling: A stage of orthodontic treatment aimed at flattening the curve of Spee for overbite reduction.

Lingual arch: A mandibular fixed anchorage reinforcing appliance, consisting of a wire soldered onto the first molar bands extending anteriorly to contact the lingual surface of the incisors, which effectively maintains arch length.

Lower anterior facial height: The soft tissue lower anterior face height is the linear distance between subnasale and gnathion. The hard tissue lower anterior facial height is the linear distance between the maxillary plane and menton.

Malocclusion: Any deviation from normal occlusion.

Moment (of a force): The tendency of a force to cause rotation.

Nance palatal arch: A maxillary fixed anchorage reinforcing appliance consisting of a wire soldered onto the first molar bands connected to an acrylic button contacting the anterior palatal surface.

Nasolabial angle: The angle between a line drawn tangent to the columella of the nose and a line connecting subnasale to the mucocutaneous border of the upper lip.

Natural head position: A standardised reproducible head position used for dento-skeletal assessment.

Non-extraction treatment: Orthodontic treatment without extraction of permanent teeth excluding the third molars.

Orthognathic surgery: Surgical repositioning of the mandible and/or maxilla for the correction of dento-facial deformity.

Osteotomy: A surgical bone cut.

Overbite: The degree of vertical overlap of the mandibular incisors by their maxillary counterparts measured perpendicular to the occlusal plane (normal = 2–4 mm) and with the teeth in occlusion.

Overjet: The horizontal distance between the labial surfaces of the mandibular incisors and the maxillary incisal edges measured parallel to the occlusal plane to the most prominent point on the maxillary central incisal edges (normal = 2–4 mm).

Paraesthesia: Reduced or abnormal sensation (e.g. tingling, burning) due to nerve damage that may occur following orthognathic surgery.

Posed smile: A voluntary smile, not linked with emotion, that is fairly reproducible (see *spontaneous smile*).

Posterior oral seal: A seal produced between the soft palate and dorsal surface of the tongue preventing open communication between the oral cavity and oropharynx.

Pre-surgical orthodontics: Orthodontic treatment carried out in preparation for orthognathic surgery.

Primate space: A naturally occurring space present mesial to the upper and distal to the lower deciduous canines.

Prognathism: A term used to describe protrusion of the maxilla and/or mandible in relationship to the cranial base.

Pubertal (adolescent) growth spurt: The acceleration in growth associated with puberty.

Quad helix appliance: A maxillary expansion appliance consisting of a stainless steel wire, incorporating four helices, attached to bands placed onto the maxillary first permanent molars.

Relapse: The return of original features of a malocclusion following treatment.

Removable appliance: An appliance that can be removed by the patient for the maintenance of oral hygiene.

Retrognathia: A term used to describe retrusion of the maxilla and/or mandible in relationship to the cranial base.

Retention: The final phase of orthodontic treatment aimed at stabilisation of corrected tooth positions.

Ricketts E-line: A line drawn tangent to the chin and nose used to assess lip fullness.

Scissor bite (lingual crossbite): Where the buccal cusps of the lower premolars/molars occlude palatal to their opposing counterparts.

Skeletal pattern: The three-dimensional relationship between the maxilla and the mandible.

Smile arc: The relationship between the curvature of the maxillary incisal edges and canine tips to the curvature of the upper border of the lower lip during the posed smile.

Spontaneous smile: An involuntary smile, linked with emotion, with maximal elevation of the upper lip (see *posed smile*).

Supernumerary teeth: Teeth in excess of the normal series.

Transseptal fibres: Periodontal fibres interconnecting adjacent teeth.

Traumatic overbite: Contact between the lower incisors and palatal mucosa that results in discomfort, inflammation, recession and/or ulceration.

Two-by-four appliance: A fixed appliance attached only to the maxillary first permanent molars (×2) and incisors (×4).

Transpalatal arch: A maxillary anchorage reinforcing appliance, consisting of a wire connecting bands placed onto the first permanent molars, that maintains the inter-molar width.

Index